The Official COVID-19 Guidebook of Published Studies, Resources, Supplements, Antivirals and TCM Herbs

Everything you wanted to know about COVID-19, but were afraid to ask

Scott Rauvers

Scott Rauvers

Get the latest Vaccine News and Updates at

www.RealNewsRevealed.com

Compiled by Master Herbalist Scott Rauvers. Founder of the Institute for Solar Studies on Behavior and Human Health

View Chapters of this book for free at

www.RealNewsRevealed.com

Copyright © by Scott Rauvers.
Second Revision. Spring 2021..

Library of Congress Catalog ISBN- 9798559015385

All rights reserved. This book or any portion thereof
may not be reproduced or used in any manner
whatsoever without the express written
permission of the publisher except for
the use of brief quotations in a
book review.

Total Number of Pages - 255

Printed in the United States of America

The Institute for Solar Studies on Human
Behavior and Health

This title is also available in Nook and Kindle versions. Just enter the title into any Internet search box to locate these versions

Other unique titles written by Scott Rauvers

- Immune System Secrets, Techniques for extending Life and surviving Pandemics

- Eternal Youth via Tao Te Ching. Longevity Secrets via Universal Energy

- The Vegetarian's Guide to Longevity via Gene Therapy and Raw Foods

- Foods, Herbs and Pharmaceuticals that Extend Lifespan. A Summary Of Over 200 Research Studies Proven To Lengthen Lifespan.

- Anti Aging Nutrition Secrets. The Fountain of Youth Seeker's Guide to Longevity

- A Centurion's Toolbox for Longevity Living Beyond 120 - 2nd Edition

- The Complete Guide to Natural Toothache Remedies and Re-mineralization

- Reverse Aging Naturally. Alchemy and Ayurveda Longevity Anti-aging Secrets

- Learn the Secrets of Prosperity and Contemplation of Your Fortune from Anywhere

Look for these unique titles at your favorite bookstore, or go online and download them immediately in Nook or Kindle editions from Amazon.com

Dedication

This book is dedicated to those brave souls on the front lines fighting COVID-19 who risk their lives each and every day, working to end the pandemic

CONTENTS

Preface.....page 14

Introduction.....page 16

Chapter 1. Common Questions and Answers about COVID-19.....page 25

Chapter 2. Vitamin D, Coffee, Honey and Nigella sativa.....page 40

Coffee may help prevent COVID-19.....What are NF-κB inhibitors?......Nigella sativa and honey reduce complications caused by COVID-19.....Why Honey may help Increase the Strength of Body's Immune System.....Vitamin D and Omega 3's.....What is a cytokine storm?.....Vitamin D Meta Data Analysis Study Involving COVID-19.....Vitamin D Synergizes with Vaccines.....Vitamin D Reduces Admissions to ICU .....Geographical Latitude and COVID-19 Cases.....Engineered Good Bacteria to help defeat COVID-19 Ivermectin .....Studies confirm COVID-19 Patients have Low Levels of Vitamin D.....Omega 3's Help Fight COVID-19.....COVID-19 Herbal Sachets.

Chapter 3. Exploring DCA, EPA and Omega 3's for the Prevention of COVID-19....page 53

How Much DHA and EPA does my body require?.....Where can I find Docosahexaenoic and Eicosapentaenoic acids?.....Where do I Obtain Omega-3s?.....Vegetarian Sources of Omega 3's.....Why the Demand for Acerola juice will soar in the coming years.....Vitamin C helps people Diagnosed with COVID-19.

Chapter 4. How Edhedra is being used for the Prevention and Treatment of COVID-19.....page 62

Ephedra for Treatment and Prevention of COVID-19.....The Amygdalus Communis Vas Formula.....Ephedra Helps Lower Cytokine Storms. The Maxing Ganshi decoction .....Ephedra for Inhibiting Influenza and Pneumonia.....Combining Ephedra with Glycyrrhiza .....What does ACE2 mean?.....Ephedrine reduces coughing.....Ephedra relieves Asthma .....The Huashi baidu Granule Formula.

Chapter 5. Chinese Herbs Scientifically Proven to Treat and Prevent COVID-19......page 71

Traditional Chinese Medicines (TCM) for treating COVID-19. .....COVID-19 Symptomology.....Herbal .formulas used for treating severe COVID-19 patients......The Maxinshigan Tang Formula .....The Baihegujin Tang Formula .....The Lian-Hua-Qing-Wen Formula.....What does IL-6, IL-8 mean?.....A Herbal Formula Recommended for the prevention and treatment of COVID-19 .....The Qingfei Paidu Decoction.....Chemical Composition of the Qingfeipaidu Decoction .....The Lianhua qingwen capsule (LH).....RECOMMENDED HERBS FOR THE EARLY STAGES OF COVID-19 INFECTION .....HERBAL FORMULAS FOR THE TREATMENT OF SEVERE COVID-19 CASES.....The 10 most commonly prescribed herbs by Chinese province.....The most frequently prescribed Herbal Combinations.....The top 10 active substances found in the most popular COVID-19 Herbal Treatments.....TCM and Western Therapy Combination Treatments.....A combination of Qingfei Paidu and Interferon .....The Shufeng Jiedu Formula.....The Qingfeipaidu decoction (QFPD).....Scutellaria baicalensis in detail.....Honeysuckle (Flos Lonicerae Japonicae) in detail.....TCM Preparations for Enhancing Immune System Functioning in Patients with COVID-19.....The Sheganmahuang decoction (SMD).....Jinhuaqinggan granules (JHQG).....Recommended Herbs for Prevention and Treatment by the Country of India (AYUSH).....Nano curcumin significantly reduces fever and cough ....Indonesian Herbs used to Fight COVID-19.....Turkish Folk Medicinal Herbs used for treating COVID-10.....A Herbal COVID-19 Resistance Formula for the Elderly. The Eight-Section Brocade.

Chapter 6. Interviews with Professional Herbalists and their recommend Herbs for Treating and Preventing COVID-19.....page 111

Plant Species.....Most Common Plants used to Treat COVID-19.....Principal Preparations.....Herbalists by Geographic Regions.....Eucalyptus Oil.....How does an Essential Oil Destroy Viruses?.....Essential Oils for Inhibiting COVID-19.....Herbs used in Steam Inhalation Therapy for combating COVID-19.....The anti-viral activity exhibited by Terpenoids .....Essential Oils that Inhibit SARS-CoV-2 .....Antiviral Essential Oils.....Citrus sp., Curcuma sp., Alpinia galanga, and Caesalpinia sappan .....Using Terpenoids to defeat COVID-19.

Chapter 7. COVID-19 Resistance Herbs.....page 121

Persian herbs .....Piper Betel .....Herbs that specifically attack SARS-CoV-2.....A list of Plants Screened for their effectiveness against COVID-19.

Chapter 8. Chinese Herbal Tablets, Capsules and Polyphenols.....page 126

My personal COVID-19 Resistance Formula.....A formula to Strengthen The Lungs.....Substances in Rhodiola rosea may promote nerve regeneration.....Echinacea.....Echinacea Recommended Dosages.....Bee Propolis ....Polyphenols for Defeating COVID-19.....Quercetin.....The Herbal Composition called Gene-Eden-VIR/Novirin .....Cinnamon.....Sang Ju Yin plus Yu Ping Feng San Protects High Risk Workers from SARS.....Astragalus.....Traditional Chinese Medicine Herbs (TCM) used for the treatment of COVID-19. Case Reviews and Recent Studies......How does Traditional Chinese Medicine (TCM) Work?.....The Qing Fei Pai Du Tang Formula.....The Qing Fei Pai Du Tang Formula.....Herbal formulas for critical patients with COVID-19 (15).....The 10 most Commonly used Herbs used to Treat COVID-19.....The Sang Ju Yin plus Yu Ping Feng San Extract.....Herbs Scientifically Proven for enhancing Lung Strength and Oxygen Capacity.....The Lian Hua Qing Wen Capsule Formula.....Traditional Chinese Medicine Herbs used for Treating Inflammation.....Traditional Chinese Medicine Herbs used for Treating Inflammation.....The Shuang Huang Lian Formula.....The Dang Gui Long Hui Pill Formula.....The Sang Ju Yin and Yu Ping Feng San Formulas.

Chapter 9. Herbs and Plants Scientifically Proven to Treat Fever, Cough, Asthma, Chronic bronchitis and the Common Cold.....page 142

Hedera helix L. - Araliaceae (Leaves).....Justicia pectoralis Jacq. (Jacq.)– Acanthaceae (Leaves).....Magnolia officinalis Rehder & E.H. Wilson - Magnoliaceae (Bark).....Mikania glomerata Spreng and M. laevigata Sch.Bip. ex Baker Asteraceae (Leaves).....Ocimum gratissimum L. -Lamiaceae (Leaves).....Salix alba L., Salix sp. - Salicaceae (Cortex) .....Zingiber officinale Roscoe - Zingiberaceae (Rhizome).....Herbs used to fight the Influenza Virus.....The Lian Hua Qing Wen Capsule Formula.....Herbs used to combat the 2003 SARS Pandemic.....The Dayuan Decoction (DYD).....The Chinese Rhubarb extract.....Herbs shown to inhibit SARS 3CLpro activity.....Escin.....Quercetin Exhibits potent Anti-Sars Activity.....Additional Herbs and Substances to reduce COVID-19 Infection .....Oleandrin.....Minerals and Vitamins for COVID-19 defense.....Vitamin K .....Vitamin C.....Selenium.....Zinc.....Elderberry Extract.....The latest studies on Chloroquine and Hydroxychloroquine for Defeating COVID-19.....How effective is Remdesevir?.....Chlorine Dioxide.....MMS is banned for commercial sale in the USA.

Chapter 10. Anti-HCoV agents active against anti-SARS-CoV activity and the common cold......page 166

Chamaecyparis obtusa (Cupressaceae) .....Betulonic acid .....Euphorbia neriifolia .....The Natural Products Guestrin, 3-theaflavin-3-gallate and Amentoflavone.

Chapter 11. Using Bald's Eyesalve to fight Antibiotic Resistant Bacteria......page 174

Chapter 12. Facts about Chlorine Dioxide......page 177

The City of Sacramento California approves the use of Chlorine Dioxide for Killing COVID-19 Germs.....Chlorine

Dioxide is Cost Effective over the Long Term.....A Chlorine Dioxide Gargle that may Kill the COVID-19 Virus..... Chlorine Dioxide is Scientifically Proven to Kill Viruses.....Dental Uses of Chlorine Dioxide in Preventing the Spread of Coronavirus (COVID-19).....Studies confirming the Virus Killing Effectiveness of Mixing Sodium Chlorite with Citric Acid.....Physical Reactions to Chlorine Dioxide .....How to Make Chlorine Dioxide.

Chapter 13. The Powerful Healing of the Natural Antibiotic Ajwain.....page 188

My Personal Experiences Using Ajwain.....Why Ajwain is a Powerful Natural Antibiotic.....Ajwain Effectively Kills numerous types of Colon Cancer Cells.....The Healing Power of Thymol.....Ajwain Oil is Fungi Toxic.....Anti-Malarial Potential of Ajwain Oil.....   A Detailed Scientific Analysis of Ajwain Seed.....Ajwain Protects Against Oxidative Stress.....Ajwain Boosts Estrogen.

Chapter 14. The Universal Healing Properties of Black Cumin Seed......page 200

Thymoquinone Protects against methionine induced hyperhomocysteinemia.....Thymoquinone is one of Nature's Most Powerful Natural Antioxidants.....Thymoquinone Protects Mammals against Diesel Exhaust Pollution.....Black Cumin Protects against Indoor Air Pollution.....Black Cumin Reduces the Side Effects of Strong Antibiotics.....Black Cumin Protects against Drug Overdose.....Black Cumin Oil Exhibits Synergy with Vitamin C.....A scientific analysis of Black Cumin Seed .....Recommended Dosage.

Chapter 15. Immune System Boosting Nutraceutical Formulas You can Make at Home.....page 210

Giloy Herbal Extract .....The Black Cumin Exercise Recovery Formula.....The Yogurt Mix Formula.....Probiotics Enhances the Immune System of the Elderly.....Vaccine and Probiotics Synergy.....How to Make The St. Germain Formula.....St. Germain Rejuvenation Synergy.....To Remove Excessive Summer Heat Stress.....The Overnight Rejuven-Essence Formula.....The Natural Probiotic Formula.

Chapter 16. Prescription Antibiotics Alter the Healthy Concentration of Stomach Microflora......page 221

SCFA's.....Do abnormalities in Healthy Stomach Microflora Contribute to Depression?.....Enhancing the Effectiveness of Antibiotics using Ultrasound.

Chapter 17. Herbal Energy Supplements You Can Make from Home......page 227

A July 2020 Study reveals that Exercise Enhances Memory.....A formula that Relaxes and Renews the Muscles.....Mega Strength Body Formula .....Neurocognition Protector Formula.....NZT. Super Neurocognition Enhancer.....A formula to Help Reduce Feelings of Depression.....A Room Temperature Probiotic that needs no refrigeration.....The Brain Food Mix.....The Carnosine Synergy Formula.....A formula for rapid Recovery from Exercise.....A formula for boosting Sexual Endurance.

Chapter 18. Understanding the link between our Brain and our Immune System.....page 242

The Placebo Effect and Knee Surgery.....Excessive Stress Contributes to Physical and Mental Illness.....The Link Between Stress and Cancer.....Gratitude has been Scientifically Proven to Strengthen the Human Immune System.....Short term stress is good for the Immune System.....How To Listen To Your Body's Subtle Messages To Enjoy Good Health.

Chapter 19. Stimulus Check Information for United States Residents....page 249

Preface

Clarity in a time of Information Overload
It is a known fact that today we live in a period of information overload, Hence excess information about COVID-19 has lead to a false anxiety and fear about the facts regarding COVID-19. Therefore this book has been purposely kept simple and factual, reducing the chance of one contracting what I term "paralysis by analysis". This book is specifically designed for the common layman seeking to gain a more deeper understanding of the COVID-19 pandemic and how to effectively protect oneself from contracting it. If you are a doctor or other medical professional specializing in TCM herbs (Traditional Chinese Medicine) for treating your patients, I have included a special chapter on herbs that have been scientifically proven effective to help prevent and treat COVID-19.

The Economic Burden from COVID-19
COVID's impact on the economy
COVID-19 is viewed as a temporary shock to economic growth, especially in developing countries. According to the Brookings Institute, compared to 2019, poverty around the world could rise by 120 million people due to the Coronavirus Pandemic. The biggest impact is most likely to be felt in India. Many people living in India have recently escaped poverty, due to strong economic growth. However as of 2020, India's per capita growth rate has steadily been in decline (to about -11 percent). This drop happens to be one of the deepest recessions in the world. Nigeria is also experiencing a deep recession, adding 85 million new people this year to its poverty. rolls.
   The reason COVID-19 is most likely to impact economically disadvantaged people the most is because many economically disadvantaged people dwell in

overcrowded accommodation. For example —7% of people defined as the poorest 20% of English households live in overcrowded housing. This presents a significant risk for the rapid spread of lower respiratory tract infections.

Secondly economically disadvantaged people are employed in occupations that do not provide a work from home option. Examples of these occupations include warehouse and supermarket workers, bus drivers and those in government services that serve the public such as police officers, ambulance workers and firemen. These occupations are also associated with increased stress and anxiety. Sudden heightened stress has been shown to weaken the human immune system; thus increasing the likleyhood of one contracting a wide range of various diseases.

References
Algren M.H., Ekholm O., Nielsen L., Ersbøll A.K., Bak C.K., Andersen P.T. Associations between perceived stress, socioeconomic status, and health-risk behaviour in deprived neighbourhoods in Denmark: a cross-sectional study. BMC Publ Health. 2018 Feb 13;18(1),

Segerstrom S.C., Miller G.E. Psychological stress and the human immune system: a meta-analytic study of 30 Years of inquiry. Psychol Bull. 2004 Jul:601-630.

Further   Reading
Poverty, inequality and COVID-19: the forgotten vulnerable. J.A. Patel. May 2020.

Introduction

Welcome to the second edition of The Official COVID-19 Guidebook of Published Studies, Resources, Supplements, Antivirals and TCM Herbs. Since the release of this first edition in 2020, many new published studies have become available, showing the best herbs and plants that help protect the body from COVID-19 as well as for treatment. Many of these new studies are by leading universities and scientific laboratories. I have included in this 2021 revised edition Essential Oils scientifically proven for Inhibiting the COVID SARS-CoV-2 virus as well as antiviral essential oils that exhibit the same effect.

It is obvious that by now most of us are all taking steps to fight COVID-19 in our own unique ways. The collective consciousness of the newly collaborating worldwide population that is working together to defeat COVID-19 is helping provide mankind a clear understanding as to why COVID-19 began. I would like to list a quote by the doctor Frank Ryan, author of *Tracking the Killer Plagues* –

> "*It serves little purpose to be scared by viruses. But it serves a good deal of purpose to understand them*"

Having authored thousands of pages on anti-aging medicine, cumulating in over a dozen books over the last decade, I began to notice that plant based medicines, unlike pharmaceuticals don't cause antibiotic resistance. Herbs and plants used to treat conditions are ecologically sound, safe and renewable, cost far less and do not need a prescription. To cite one example, I show in this book the herb Ajwain is as effective as some antibiotics. Also I would like to point out that many substances that are anti-malarial, anti-HIV and anti-cancer have been shown to have potential for the treatment and prevention of COVID-19.

Over the course of thousands of years, plants have learned how to deal with viruses in such a way that they naturally build up a resistance to them. This is because a plant can't just pack up and move to avoid a virus, it has to stay put and learn to make the ideal chemistry necessary for its survival.

The Surprise Arrival of COVID-19
Being a writer, I have had the opportunity to connect with people from all walks of life. At the start of the pandemic, many government officials stated things would "get back to normal" within about 8 months. As Thanksgiving approaches, when I think about that statement I feel myself cringe. Being a published science nutrition writer, keeping up to date with all the latest, knew what we considered "*normal*" was not going to occur anytime soon for the vast majority of us.

It is painfully obvious (*no pun intended*) that many state and federal agencies were totally ill-prepared to handle a pandemic of such epic proportions. This has resulted in, many unanswered questions about COVID-19, leaving a huge gap in our understanding as the pandemic rages on. We have all witnessed how the World Health Organization has handled the pandemic due to the numerous political pressures placed upon it. People with chronic disease and the elderly are the groups most at risk for contracting

COVID-19. It is a sad unfortunate fact that some COVID-19 deaths were the result of systematic government misconduct The unfortunate death of these people should not be regarded as a mere statistic used to argue differences between nations. A person who has died of COVID-19 in New York is just as important as a person who died in Wuhan China. We should remain aware about COVID-19 becoming an exercise towards radical de-humanisation.

My Background and Qualifications
My writing skills were honed as a student studying writing at Weber State University in Utah with my anti-aging research and publishing from studying Gerontology (the science of aging) also at Weber. On December 11th, 2020 I published a short article on my website about the shortcomings of the COVID-19 vaccine, why it was rushed and questioned its safety. I specifically stated that the virus would mutate in the coming months as the vaccine was rolled out. It just so happened that on Jan. 3, 2021 the first reported mutation of the COVID-19 virus was discovered in Minnesota USA and is expected to soon be the main dominant virus in the United States. I don't state this fact to brag, but to let the reader know that I am able to follow the data and information faithfully and write about it factually.

Secondly, I would like to make clear that I am not a doctor or medical practitioner. My knowledge of healing and herbs stems from the past 10 years of researching and using anti-aging herbal formulas and longevity extracts. This experience has taught me to interpret the data in scientific published studies and associated literature and make it easy for anyone to understand the information.

Many of us have felt frustrated when reading a published paper and are sometimes confused as to the terminology used. This book is simply an interpretation of the latest published studies on COVID-19 as they relate to herbal medicine, along with a few of my own popular energy and immune system boosting formulas included along the way. Hence, you could spend days or months seeking the latest and best information on plants and herbs that fight COVID-19 and not understand the terms used. Hence, this book has done all the work for you, saving you countless hours of time and frustration. Keep this book as a reference for when the next pandemic strikes, which is inevitable and you will not be caught unaware.

In summary, the purpose of this book is to give to you the very best information on broad-spectrum systematic antiviral herbs that have been scientifically proven to be very effective COVID-19 viral infections, as well as herbs for treating influenza and pummenoia. Many of these plants and herbs can be easily obtained and can be grown in your own backyard or in a kitchen garden. They can also be made into Tinctures / Extracts allowing you to use far less, making them last for years. For those of you new to extracts I have written a book on how anyone can make their own extracts at home. The book is called The Official Guidebook of How to Make Tinctures and Alchemy Spagyric Formulas and thankfully has received a good rating from my fans over the years.

Today many researchers around the globe, especially in mainland China, have been forced to come to the realization and understanding that some antiviral herbs are more effective than some prescription antibiotics, especially when a change of lifestyle is added (*reduction in stress and a moderate change in diet*). This new "green gold rush" has resulted in many labs, both corporate and academic, to identify the most potent herbs and plants, their ideal growing conditions and how best to prepare them.

We as a human race need to embrace this new paradigm of ecologically friendly healing, because the technology to make this a reality is now only just becoming economically viable. As nature inspires and motivates us, common sense tells us that this new paradigm is not just human friendly, but helps us to more clearly connect with each other on a global level.

Humanity is at a cross roads. We as a species have the opportunity to create something new, where we can more perfectly regain our health and heal the earth in the process. I believe that this is one important clue as to why COVID-19 began in the first place; to teach humanity to work together for the first time on a global scale.

It is my sincere wish that you find the material revealed to you in these pages stimulating to your thinking......allowing you to step outside the box of traditional mainstream medicine.

Scott Rauvers

Author

Plant Based Medicine is gaining widespread recognition
Research is discovering what herbalists have known for centuries, that plants are an important source of substances for defeating many types of viruses and bad bacteria. In North America, The Andrew Weil Center for Integrative Medicine recommends the polyphenol-rich plants such as licorice herb, onions, apples, chamomille, Chinese skullcap, tomatoes, oranges, nuts, berries, turmeric root, green tea, parsley and celery in order to reduce the risk of infection (*Alschuler et al., 2020*).

Several studies in 2020 have been published researching the best plants and herbs to defeat COVID-19; some of which may serve as leads for developing new drugs. The details of some of the studies below will be shared in greater detail later on in this book -

Natural products for COVID-19 prevention and treatment regarding to previous coronavirus infections and novel studies. Boozari, M et al. Phyther. Res. 2020.

Natural products and their derivatives against coronavirus: A review of the non-clinical and pre-clinical data. Islam, M.T. et al. Phyther. Res. 2020, 34, 2471–2492.

Traditional Chinese medicine in the treatment of patients infected with 2019-new coronavirus (SARS-CoV-2): A review and perspective. Yang, Y. et al. Int. J. Biol. Sci. 2020, 16, 1708–1717.

Antiviral and Immunomodulatory Effects of Phytochemicals from Honey against COVID-19: Potential mechanisms of action and future Directions. Al-Hatamleh et al. Molecules 2020, 25, 5017.

The development of Coronavirus 3C-Like protease (3CLpro) inhibitors from 2010 to 2020. Liu, Y et al. Eur. J. Med. Chem. 2020, 206, 112711.

Discovering small-molecule therapeutics against SARS-CoV-2. Tiwari, V et al. Drug Discov. Today 2020, 25, 1535-1544.

Current Findings Regarding Natural Components with Potential. Zhou, J et al. Anti-2019-nCoVActivity. Front. CellDev.Biol. 2020, 8, 589.

Natural products' role against COVID-19. da Silva Antonio, et al. . RSC Adv. 2020, 10, 23379-23393.

Screening for natural and derived bio-active compounds in preclinical and clinical studies: One of the frontlines of fighting the coronaviruses pandemic. Khalifa, S.A.M et al. Phytomedicine 2020, 153311.

Anti-SARS-CoV Natural Products with the Potential to Inhibit SARS-CoV-2 (COVID-19). Verma, S et al. Front. Pharmacol. 2020, 11, 561334.

Potential roles of medicinal plants for the treatment of viral diseases focusing on COVID-19: A review. Adhikari, B et al. Phyther. Res. 2020.

Natural Products and Natural-Product-Inspired Chemicals as Potential Counters to SARS-CoV-2 Infection. Wang, Z et al. Front. Pharmacol. 2020, 11, 1013.

Traditional Chinese herbal medicine for treating novel coronavirus (COVID-19) pneumonia: protocol for a systematic review and meta-analysis. Zhang, Y., et al. (2020). Syst. Rev. 9, 1-6. doi: 10.1186/s13643-020-01343-4

In the News: Coronavirus and "Alternative" Treatment *(National Institute of Health). Available at:* https://www.nccih.nih.gov/health/in-thenews-coronavirus-and-alternative-treatments. NIH (2020).

Dietary therapy and herbal medicine for COVID-19 prevention: A review and perspective. Panyod, S., Ho, C.-T., and Sheen, L.-Y. (2020).

Challenges at the Time of COVID-19: Opportunities and Innovations in Antivirals from Nature. Planta Med. 86, 659-664. doi: 10.1055/a-1177-4396. Hempel, G., et al. (2020)

Herbal medicine and pattern identification for treating COVID-19: a rapid review of guidelines. Integr. Med. Res. 9, 100407. doi: 10.1016/j.imr.2020.100407. Lee, M. S. et al. (2020a).

It is from the above information that Official Chinese TCM Prescriptions recommended for the Treatment and Diagnosis of COVID-19 were developed. These are the following and will be reviewed in detail in this book - The Qingfei Paidu decoction (QFPDD), The Maxing Shigan decoction (MXSGD), The Shufeng Jiedu formula (SFJD), Lianhua Qingwen capsules (LHQW), Huoxiang Zhengqi capsules (HXZQ), The Dayuan decoction (DYD), The Huashi Baidu formula (HSBD), The Huashi Baidu formula (HSBD) and Jinhua Qinggan granules (JHQG).

Reference
Research progress of traditional Chinese medicine against COVID-19. Wei Ren et al. February 2021.

Herbal Advisory
For those of you using herbs and their associated formulas, it can help to keep a diary of the herbs (or medication) that you are taking in order to inform doctors and other health care professionals in the rare case you or a loved one are hospitalized.

Anesthesia and Herbs
Research has documented that herbal medicines interact with anesthesia (*Levy et al., 2017; AANA, 2020*). Hence anesthesiologists advise against taking the following herbs before surgery or other medical procedures -

• Echinacea - theorized to increase the risk of liver damage

• Ginkgo, St. John's wort and valerian - may increase the effects of anesthesia and make it harder to wake-up. They may also cause irregular heart rhythms.

• Ginseng, licorice and milk thistle - may cause a rapid heart rate and high blood pressure

• Garlic, ginkgo, green tea, ginger, Saw palmetto and feverfew - may cause prolonged bleeding. Garlic may increase the effects of some pain relievers.

Chapter 1. Common Questions and Answers about COVID-19

When was the first case of COVID-19 reported?
The first case of Coronavirus was officially reported on December 30, 2019, in the city of Wuhan, Hubei province, China [1]. A few months later on March 11, 2020 the SARS-CoV-2 virus (*now officially COVID-19*) was declared as a global pandemic by World Health Organization (*K. Kumari et al. 2020*).

What is the current Relapse Rate of COVID-19?
Statistically speaking the total rate of relapse is 0.1 % of 8000 cases. As of 2021, no published data exists stating relapses have occurred in many hospitals.

How similar is SARS-CoV to COVID-19?
The coronavirus shares a 79.5% sequence identity with SARS-CoV (*Stoermer M. Feb 2020*). SARS-CoV is the virus that became a regional pandemic in China between 2002 and 2003. Similarities exist in the symptoms between COVID-19 and SARS with COVID-19 mainly targeting the lower airway region of the chest, possibly due to the COVID-19 virus being so small. SARS-CoV-2 results in inflammatory and immune system responses, leading to cytokine storms. Pathological observations have discovered inflammation can take place in the early stages COVID-19 pneumonia. Hence, effective potent anti-inflammatory and antiviral herbs and drugs are recommended for COVID-19 patients that show signs of pneumonia.

Does SARS-CoV cause COVID-19?
SARS-CoV has a high level of sequence identity to SARS-

CoV-2. SARS-CoV-2 is the agent that causes COVID-19. This is why many researchers use the SARS-CoV during their research to find cures for COVID-19.

Where did the COVID-19 virus first originate?
While there is no evidence of the direct cause of COVID-19, scientists looking for the origin of SARS-CoV-2 and its related animal-to-human transmission stated in a recent research study published in February 2021 stated a Thai cave that housed bats had a single isolate (named RacCS203) that was most likely related to the RmYN02 isolate found in Rhinolophus malayanus in Yunnan, China. The bats also exhibited SARS-CoV-2 neutralizing antibodies as well as bats at a wildlife checkpoint in Southern Thailand. In summary the discovery of the isolate (RaTG13 bat coronavirus) in China suggests a high probability that the virus first manifested itself inside bats that live in caves.

Further Reading
Evidence for SARS-CoV-2 related coronaviruses circulating in bats and pangolins in Southeast Asia Supaporn Wacharapluesadee. Chee Wah Tan et al.

Which 4 countries have the lowest death count from COVID-19?
According to John Hopkins, as of November 2020, the countries with the lowest numbers of deaths are - Papua New Guinea, Iceland, New Zealand and Vietnam. These are the places to be if you want to ride out the pandemic over the long term.
It is interesting to note here that a nasal spray that is derived from New Zealand algae may in the future be used as a preventive measure for COVID-19. The algae has been shown to be effective against hepatitis, Ebola and herpes as

well as a broad spectrum of coronaviruses, including MERS and SARS. The research team originally used the algae as a preventive for human immunodeficiency virus (HIV). Because COVID-19 typically enters through the nostrils and the mouth, the nasal spray makes it an excellent preventive, stopping COVID-19 from infecting the lungs. This algae also has an affinity for coronaviruses' surfaces, which means it does not affect healthy cells. Scientists are making the molecule known as Q-griffithsin by using an anti-viral protein that is abundant in the New Zealand red algae Griffithsia and Nicotiana benthamiana; a species that is part of the tobacco family. The nasal spray would be used for high risk people such as emergency medical service workers and health care workers. Because Q-griffithsin exhibits broad spectrum activity it may be useful in the future to treat future pandemics [1a] [1b].

Do Lockdowns Reduce Deaths?
A study found that deaths of all kinds sharply dropped after a lockdown, with the largest drop in traffic deaths. Suicide and homicide rates also dropped [1c].

How does a COVID-19 virus infection affect a person who becomes infected with COVID-19?
The infection begins at the body's respiratory region, resulting in a mild respiratory tract infection. In professional medical terms this is known as the 'severinfee acute respiratory syndrome'. This is rapidly followed by respiratory failure, shock and finally multiple organ failure [2] [3]. These symptoms may be accompanied by diarrhea, headache, lymphopenia and fatigue, (*Rothan and Byrareddy, 2020*). In certain cases a high incidence of cardiovascular symptoms may accompany the infection (*Zheng et al., 2020*). Elderly people or those with medical problems such as

diabetes, chronic respiratory disease, cardiovascular disease and cancer are more likely to develop more severe forms of illness if they become infected with the COVID-19 virus (*WHO, 2020a*).

What does the Coronavirus Look Like?
The Coronavirus lives inside an RNA viruses (*composed of single stranded RNA*). This strand is reported to be one of the longest RNA viruses and acts as an RNA messenger. It is spherical in shape (*approx. 125nm diameter*). The exterior consists of club-shaped spike-proteins which stick out from its surface, resulting in a crown-like appearance of sphere (*Lu et al., 2020*) [4].

Are Chinese Herbs Superior to Conventional Western Therapy?
A research study discovered that TCM herbs (Traditional Chinese Medicine) in combination with conventional western therapy exhibited a more significant effect compared to conventional western therapy for reducing the aggravation rate for non-serious patients. For the duration of fever, a study (*Wang et al., 2020c*) found that the group taking TCM medicine exhibited significant improvements in a reduction of their fever ($p = 0.035$) compared to the control group [4a].

What are the most popular herbs being used in China today to treat COVID-19 patients?
At the very start of the pandemic, Traditional Chinese Medicinal herbs (TCMH) and their respective formulas and associated treatments were used in 91.50% of COVID-19 cases in China [4b]. Out of 179 single herbal formulas used for treating COVID-19 in China, the most frequently used herbs at the time were Glycyrrhizae Radix et Rhizome, Scutellariae Radix and Armeniacae Semen Amarum. The

main substances that were most active in the herbs were quercetin, β-sitosterol and stigmasterol. The study concluded that 10 new herbal formulas emerged from this group as being potentially useful for combating COVID-19. The medicinal properties of the herbs were as follows -

Antipyretic (47%)

Expectorant and cough-suppressing (22%)

Dampness-resolving (21%)

Later on in this book I specifically target herbs and their associated combinations that have been scientifically proven to exhibit a 90%+ or better success rate at treating COVID-19 patients. This is especially relevant information as effectiveness of the COVID-19 vaccine continues to erode due to the ever emerging variants of the COVID-19 virus (mutations).

What Percentage of People in China are receiving TCM based Treatments and How Effective are they?
The rate of TCM treatment for patients of COVID-19 in China was 87 %. The total effectiveness of treatment was 92 %. Only 5% of patients have shown worse symptoms (*Yang et al., 2020a*).

A more recent study published in February of 2021 titled: *Review on the potential action mechanisms of Chinese medicines in treating Coronavirus Disease*, that was conducted by Y.F. Huang and colleagues states that the total effective rate is now over 90 %..

Traditional Chinese Medicine treatments (TCM) have so far shown to be superior in preventing infected COVID-19 patients who have severe cases of COVID-19 and has reduced the number of patients admitted to an ICU. In the

Jin-Chang Hospital in China, with an efficacy rate of TCM treatment showing an effectiveness of almost 100% (99.2%). Clinical experience and scientific basis (*David Y.W. Lee et al. Sept 2020*).

When was the Gene Sequence of COVID-19 first de-coded?
It was on January 10 of 2020 that the Chinese Center for Disease Control and Prevention released the whole gene sequence of the COVID-19 virus to the World Health Organization (*China-CDC, 2020*). It was on January 29, 2020 that Chinese scientists reported the completion of the genome sequence of COVID-19 (*Lu et al., 2020*).

Does the COVID-19 Pandemic Increase my chance of becoming depressed?
COVID-19 Increases Susceptibility to Depression
A study published in JAMA Network Open (by Boston University Researchers) [4c] found that COVID-19 tripled the rate of depression in the United States; in all demographic groups. Those with financial worries were especially hard hit. The study looked at 1,441 respondents from Mar 31st to Apr 13 in 2020. This was when 96% of United States was under coronavirus-related lockdowns. Researchers found that 27.8% of adults reported depression during 2020, compared with just 8.5% before the COVID-19 pandemic. Before the pandemic began, 10.1% of women reported being depressed and 6.9% of men. During the pandemic 22.2% of women reported being depressed and 21.9% of men. Those most at risk were those living with a partner (37.7%) and those who never married (39.8%). People who were married were only 18.3% depressed compared to those who were widowed, divorced, or separated (31.5%). The authors also stated mental illness will grow over time, particularly among at-risk populations.

How is COVID-19 Transmitted?
The COVID-19 virus is spread via droplets that consist of the coronavirus when a person coughs, sneezes, or breathes in the surrounding region. These particles float in the air and adhere to surfaces which your hands than touch the eyes, nose, or mouth regions of the body. If the body is susceptible to the virus, than within 2 to 14 days, the immune system will take steps to respond via coughing, difficulty breathing, chills, fever and muscle pains. It can also include a loss of taste and smell. Because the virus is so small, it is very prone to airborne dispersion. The virus may be spreading through tiny aerosol particles which penetrate deep into the lungs. This in turn triggers severe respiratory infections. Because these tiny particles reach into the deepest regions of the body, they can also affect the internal organs.

As a person enters the asymptomatic phase of COVID-19, it becomes highly contagious with a 44 % transmission rate before symptoms begin appearing in a person [3a]. Recent studies have also found COVID-19 may be spreading by feces [3b].

The 4 Symptomatic Stages of COVID-19 are [3c] -

1- Early stages. Symptoms include cold-dampness attacking the lung and spleen.

2 - Middle Stage. Symptoms include of cold-dampness blocking the energy of the lung and spleen.

3 - Late stage. Symptoms include cold-dampness injuring the spleen and shutting down the lungs.

4 - Recovery stage. Symptoms include qi-deficiency of lung and spleen.

How soon will a vaccine be 100% effective?
At this time 18 vaccine projects are currently in full operation. In times past, even the fastest vaccination programs took a minimum of four years and that was when the pandemic(s) were not global in scope. Current estimates state it may take anywhere from 6 months to a full year to complete a full clinical evaluation of how effective new vaccines are. With the introduction of the mutation (variant) of the virus constantly resurfacing in other countries, this could cause a delay in the vaccine's clinical evaluation process.

How Effective are Herbs for Treatment of COVID-19?
Herbal remedies may seem harmless; however if they are misused, they may increase a person's risk for COVID-19. The latest data is starting to show that certain herbs are effective in treating and preventing COVID-19 for some people, and not for others. To date, there is not enough data regarding the use of herbal remedies for the novel coronavirus. Effectiveness of herbs may vary due to lifestyle, diet and other factors.

Why should I incorporate herbs into my COVID-19 defense strategy?
With the recent Opioid Epidemic in the United States, more and more people are starting to trust herbal medications for treating various ailments. While the new vaccines may not themselves be addictive, some prescription medication for treating COVID-19 may end up being addictive. Hence, herbs are the best route for recovery from COVID-19 as they become rarely addictive.

Which 2 countries have the highest death count from COVID-19?
According to John Hopkins, as of November 5th, 2020, the U.S. and Brazil are the leaders in the numbers of deaths from COVID-19.

What are the symptoms of COVID-19?
Persons exposed to COVID-19 and that come down with the infection can experience anywhere from mild symptoms to severe illness; depending upon various factors such as immune system strength, health status and age. Symptoms typically appear between 2 and 14 days after exposure. If you experience any of the following, you may have COVID-19 and are strongly urged to seek medical attention immediately -

- *Muscle or body aches*
- *Sudden loss of taste or smell*
- *Headache*
- *Fever or chills*
- *Shortness of breath or difficulty breathing*
- *Nausea or vomiting*
- *Sudden unexpected Fatigue*
- *Sore throat*
- *Diarrhea*

How do I Avoid Prone Risk Areas?
Research is just starting to show that people who live in cities where people are closely packed together have shown the most increase in COVId-19 cases. New York City for example is one such case.

According to a Time Magazine Article titled-

Europe's Second Wave of COVID-19 is Being Driven by Two Countries, that was published on October 27th, 2020. -

the article states that as of Oct 23rd, 2020, the country of Belgium is the epicenter of the European Union's second COVID-19 wave; having the continent's highest per-capita number of cases (*besides Andorra*). Belgium also has the world's third highest number of COVID-19 deaths after Peru and San Marino. The Czech Republic also shows above numbers of COVID-19 cases.

Belgium and the Czech Republic have relatively high population densities. Basically Belgium is one big city and in Brussels the population density is particularly high. For example, for every kilometer of land in Belgium there exist on average 377 people. In the Czech Republic the number is approximately 137 people per square kilometer.

The Time Magazine article goes on to state that COVID-19 is spread by students returning home from school on the weekends; exposing the infection to their parents. According to Jan Pačes, virologist from the Czech Academy of Sciences, cases of COVID-19 soared shortly after schools reopened on Sept. 1, 2020; with the majority of new cases occurring in young people and eventually reaching higher ages. Jan Pačes goes on to state that an estimated 30% of new COVID-19 infections came from people associating in their homes.

Do Face Masks Really Work? What does the CDC say? The CDC states that associating with a person diagnosed with COVID-19 for longer than 15 minutes may cause one to contract COVID-19 whether a face mask is worn or not. The CDC goes on to state that masks "may" help some people infected with COVID-19 from spreading the virus, and add "there is less information" if masks can effectively protect a person coming into contact with someone who has COVID-

19. In Belgium and Spain authorities have made mask wearing mandatory, however their infection numbers have still risen.

In May 2020 the CDC released a meta-analysis study involving 14 controlled, extended trials that studied the effects of mask usage. The study discovered that no reduction took place in the rate of laboratory-confirmed cases of influenza, which is a respiratory illness similar to COVID-19.

Who is most at risk for contracting COVID-19?
On average 1 in 5 people diagnosed with COVID-19 will require some type of intensive care. Recent studies have found that person's diagnosed with hypertension and diabetes are more at risk for death from COVID-19 [5].

COVID-19 Risk Group
Coronavirus can be a killer. Or to others, no big deal. It puts some in intensive care, or with others, comes and goes on others without leaving a mark, more rumor than reality. As of October 1st, 2020 1 million people have died globally from COVID-19.

QUICK FACTS
COVID-19 affects more people over the age of 60 and those diagnosed with chronic conditions such as diabetes, obesity, lung disease, hypertension and heart disease.

The average age for people who die from COVID 19 in northern Italy is 81 and in England there has been virtually no major deaths of COVID-19 for people under the of 45.

Obesity Increases One's Chance Of Contracting COVID-19
Jennifer Lighter, hospital epidemiologist at NYU Langone, stated in her research report that obesity is the number 1 factor among people below age 60 who contract COVID-19 and that patients diagnosed with COVID-19 that have a body mass index of between 30 and 34 were twice as more likely to contract COVID-19 compared to patients with a BMI under 30. Also patients with a BMI index of 35+ were three times more likely to die from COVID-19.

Numerous research papers have tried to see if different strains of the virus are more lethal. One strain, which is popular in Europe and the United States has a genetic mutation that affects the spike protein. This structure lets the virus bind to receptor cells in humans. European scientists stated in a study that variations exist on two places in the human genome which can cause respiratory failure in COVID-19 patients in Italy and Spain. Patients with Type A blood showed a 50% higher risk of needing ventilator assistance, due to these people being more susceptible to inflammation. Type O people however showed a partial protective effect. People with Type A's are more susceptible to blood clots and may be more at risk for severe COVID-19 cases.

Summary
If you are over 60, or overweight, take extra measures to protect yourself. And if you are not in this category, taking measures to keep your immune system strong such as though exercise, specific herbs, along with wearing a face mask and the through washing of hands will greatly reduce your chances of contracting COVID-19. These are all common sense precautions that anyone who wants to avoid the COVID-19 infection should take.

Why should I buy this book?

As the vaccine's effectiveness continues to be eroded by the ever-emerging variants (mutated forms of COVID-19) specific herbs and plants scientifically proven to help defeat COVID-19 may be the best defense strategy to help cope with COVID-19. Once the pandemic is over, the information in this book will be invaluable to help one stay healthy during future pandemics, which are inevitable. Take this book to a reputable herbalist and show him or her the herbal formulas if you don't feel comfortable mixing these herbs yourself or lack access to any of them.

Another key reason to keep this book for future reference, is if in the event that civilization collapses and the infrastructure necessary to make vaccines no longer exists, plants and herbs will still be readily available.

Numbered References. Chapter 1

(1) X. Xu, et al., Evolution of the novel coronavirus from the ongoing Wuhan outbreak and modeling of its spike protein for risk of human transmission, Sci. China Life Sci. 63 (3) (2020) 457-460, doi:10.1007/s11427-020-1637-5).

(1a) Griffithsin, a Highly Potent Broad-Spectrum Antiviral Lectin from Red Algae: From Discovery to Clinical Application. Choongho Lee. Oct 2019.

(1b) Formula Developed to Combat HIV Could Work as Novel Coronavirus Preventive. Amerigo Allegretto. April 2020. https://www.pittwire.pitt.edu/news/formula-developed-combat-hiv-could-double-novel-coronavirus-preventive.

(1c) Impact of COVID-19 lockdown policy on homicide, suicide, and motor vehicle deaths in Peru. Renzo J.C. Calderon-Anyosa and Jay S. Kaufman. Nov 2020.

(2) X. Xu, et al., Evolution of the novel coronavirus from the ongoing Wuhan outbreak and modeling of its spike protein for risk of human transmission, Sci. China Life Sci. 63 (3) (2020) 457-460, doi:10.1007/s11427-020-1637-5).

(3) Bai et al., 2020; Zhou et al., 2020.

(3a) H. Luo, M. Zhao, D. Tan, C. Liu, L. Yang, L. Qiu, Y. Gao, H. Yu, Anti-COVID-19 drug screening: frontier concepts and core technologies, Chin. Med. 15 (1) (2020).

(3b) W. Wang, Y. Xu, R. Gao, R. Lu, K. Han, G. Wu, W. Tan, Detection of SARS-CoV-2 in different types of clinical specimens, JAMA. 323 (18) (2020) 1843–1844.

(3c) Research progress of traditional Chinese medicine against COVID-19. Wei Ren et al. February 2021.

(4) Natural and Nature-Derived Products Targeting Human Coronaviruses. Konstantina Vougogiannopoulou et al. Jan 2021. Department of Pharmacognosy and Natural Products Chemistry, Faculty of Pharmacy, National and Kapodistrian University of Athens, Panepistimiopolis Zografou, 15771 Athens, Greece.

(4a) Chinese Herbal Medicine Used With or Without Conventional Western Therapy for COVID-19: An Evidence Review of Clinical Studies. www.frontiersin.orgShi-Bing Liang. et al. Feb 2021.

(4b) Analysis on herbal medicines utilized for treatment of COVID-19. Lu Luoa. et al .July 2020.

(4c) Online report. Depression triples in US adults amid COVID-19 stressors. September 2020.

(5) Guan W., Liang W., Zhao Y., Liang H., Chen Z., Li Y. Comorbidity and its impact on 1590 patients with covid-19 in China: a nationwide analysis. Eur Respir J. 2020 Mar 26;55(5).

Chapter 2. Vitamin D, Coffee, Honey and Nigella sativa.

Before I share the herbs that help treat COVID-19, I would first like to point out that one of the most popular western beverages has shown potential to help protect one against the COVID-19 virus.

Coffee may help prevent COVID-19
Parthenolide and Caffeic acid phenethyl ester (CAPE) are both found in coffee. These have been discovered to significantly decrease the levels of proinflammatory cytokines and lung infection in mice infected with SARS. Parthenolide and caffeic acid phenylethyl ether (CAPE) are both NF-κB inhibitors. The study showed that treatment with drugs that inhibit NF-κB activation can lead to reductions in inflammation and lung pathology in SARS-CoV-infected cultured cells as well as mice. It has also been shown to significantly increase the survival of mice after they were infected with SARS-CoV [1].

What are NF-κB inhibitors?
The human immune system is a complex organism. NF-κB is a regulation of inflammatory responses and is responsible for returning balance to various pro-inflammatory genes that make up immune cells. This in turn regulates the activation and better functioning of the body's inflammatory T cells.

In a research paper published in October 2020 titled: *Caffeine and caffeine-containing pharmaceuticals as promising inhibitors for 3-chymotrypsin-like protease of SARS-CoV-2* that was conducted by Amin O. Elzupir and colleagues, it states that linagliptin and caffeine are recommended for COVID-19 treatment after in vitro, in vivo and clinical trial validation. The paper also stated that the seven drugs: linagliptin, caffeine, theophylline, dyphylline, pentoxifylline, bromotheophylline and istradefylline show potential for treating COVID-19 due to their binding affinity to 3CLpro of His41 and Cys145.

Summary
The activation of NF-κB signaling pathway exhibits a major contribution to reducing inflammation caused by SARS-CoV infections. Also NF-κB inhibitors exist as promising antivirals in helping treat infections caused by SARS-CoV activity as well as other pathogenic human coronaviruses. Substances that directly target host cells components may be helping reduce SARS-CoV-2 infection. The natural products β-sitosterol, betulinic acid, cholesterol, hopane and glycyrrhizin may reduce SARS-CoV-2 by the direction action of the inhibition of the attachment of the virus (*which is lipid-dependent*) to host cells.
    A study by Chowdhary et al. (*2003*) discovered anticancer and antiretroviral activities of Betulinic acid, which is a pentacyclic triterpenoid extracted from the bark of the white Betula alba var. pubescens tree (*Thurnher et al., 2003*) [2].

Nigella sativa and honey reduce complications caused by COVID-19
Later in this book, I devote an entire chapter to Nigella sativa, however here I would like to point out a recent study published in 2021 titled: *Efficacy of honey and Nigella sativa against COVID-19: HNS-COVID-PK Trial*, that was funded by the Smile Welfare Organization and conducted by Shaikh Zayed and colleagues at the Medical Complex and Services Institute of Medical Sciences (NIH Clinical Trial Register number: NCT04347382), the stated that a mullticenter-

randomized-controlled-trial involving 313 patients that were diagnosed with COVID-19 that received a Nigella sativa and Honey combination for up to 2 weeks (some of the patients were placebo) exhibited a reduction in their symptoms as well as a reduction in 30-day mortality. The researchers also found that the Nigella sativa and Honey combination reduced symptoms in COVID-19 patients after 7 days (in moderate and severe cases) and found that the Nigella sativa and Honey combination cleared the virus after approximately 4 days in moderate and severe cases. After 6 days 63.6% of the patients were returning to normal activities in moderate cases and 28% in severe cases. Overall a reduction in 30-day mortality among severe patients was shown when they took the Nigella sativa and Honey combination. No adverse side effects were reported by any of the patients. The researchers of the study concluded that a combination of Nigella sativa and Honey is safe to use alone or in combination with other treatments in order to reduce or eliminate the effects of COVID-19.

Currently an ongoing clinical trial titled: *Prospects of honey in fighting against COVID-19: pharmacological insights and therapeutic promises* is being conducted by Khandkar Shaharina Hossain and colleagues with hopes to establish a relationship with honey for the treatment of COVID-19 due to the fact that honey may be beneficial for COVID-19 patients by boosting the body's immune system by exhibiting antiviral activities.

Why Honey may help Increase the Strength of Body's Immune System
Honey is a natural antiviral and bee propolis is rich in bioactive compounds that exhibit powerful natural anti-inflammatory, antimicrobial, bactericidal, immunomodulatory and antioxidant activities. A study reviewed these for use as adjuvant treatments for people

infected with severe acute respiratory syndrome-coronavirus-2 (SARS-CoV-2). Computer molecular simulations state that flavonoids in honey and propolis (caffeic acid phenyl ester, naringin, rutin, luteolin and artepillin C) may help reduce cytokine storms and viral replication. Also propolis ethanolic extract, and propolis liposomes have exhibited similar activity to the potent antiviral drug remdesivir. Rutin has been shown to help reduce the SARS-CoV-2 virus (in vitro) and along with naringin, inhibit SARS-CoV-2 infection (in Vero E6 cells). The review also states that hospitalized COVID-19 patients that received green Brazilian propolis or a combination of honey and Nigella sativa exhibited early recovery from their symptoms as well as an earlier discharge from the hospital and less mortality than COVID-19 patients that received standard care and that propolis extracts delivered by nanocarriers exhibit better antiviral effects against SARS-CoV-2 than ethanolic extracts [2a].

Stevia Extract
Stevia is used as an alternative to sugar to sweeten foods and drinks. A study found that extracts of Stevia exhibited showed virostatic and virucidal activity against 229E [3].

Vitamin D and Omega 3's
Vitamin D, as well as Omega 3's have shown great promise in treating as well as acting as a natural preventative against contracting COVID-19. A research study concluded that a healthy intake of vitamin D helped strengthen the immune system by reducing the risk for the body to generate a cytokine storm in response to a COVID-19 infection. The study concluded that improving vitamin D status in the general population, especially in patients hospitalized with COVID-19, may be of benefit in reducing

the severity of deaths from people diagnosed with COVID-19 [4].

What is a cytokine storm?

A cytokine storm is an "*overreaction*" to an infection in the body. This causes the immune system to overproduce cytokines and excess immune system cells in order to fight infection. It as if the body's immune system shifts into overdrive, which is why only small amounts work very well in substances that produce cytokine storms. Excessive cytokine storms can cause damage to the lungs and are suspected to play a role in some cases of severe COVID-19 (*Mehta, Lancet 2020*). To put this in plain english, the body's immune system becomes over reactive and puts out above average levels of energy in order to fight the COVID-19 virus. Cytokine storms have come to be the second leading cause of death in COVID-19 patients [5]. Recent studies confirm that injuries of multiple organs in the body caused by the COVID-19 virus may be related to Cytokine Storms which lead to an accumulation of oxidative stress-free radicals in the body [6]

Further Reading
COVID-19: consider cytokine storm syndromes and immunosuppression. Puja Mehta.

Simple facts about Vitamin D
Vitamin D is a vitamin which is lipid-soluble. It is essential for strong bones. It is produced in the skin via sunlight or from foods such as Cod Liver Oil and some types of fish. Lately some food manufacturers have started adding vitamin D to food such as orange juice (fortified).

Vitamin D plays an important role in Immune System Functioning

Vitamin D has been shown to regulate the adaptive and innate immune response of the immune system (*Rosen et al., 2016*) and demonstrate the ability to destroy bad viruses, including the HCV genotype infection [7]. It has also exhibited antiviral activity as elucidated by Grant et al. (*2020*). Another study discovered that Vitamin D showed effectiveness in reducing the hazards associated with viral pandemics [8].

Studies suggest people with low levels of vitamin D are more likely to test positive for COVID-19, as well as have more severe symptoms. A Singapore study involving older men and women who had contracted COVID-19 found that those who took Vitamin D along with magnesium and vitamin B12, that within only one day of COVID-19 hospitalization, they were much less likely to require oxygen therapy and / or intensive care compared to the group that did not take the Vitamin D/magnesium/vitamin B12 combo. Magnesium has been shown to enhance the immune system by boosting the body's T-and helper cells (*Liang et al., 2012*) as well as help ward off viral infections [51] (*Chaigne-Delalande et al., 2013*).

Vitamin D Meta Data Analysis Study Involving COVID-19

A research study titled: *Effects of Vitamin D on COVID-19 Infection and Prognosis: A Systematic Review*. that was published in 2021 by Hiwot Yisak and colleagues, looked at a total of 1,005,042 COVID-19 patients from 20 European countries and their associated studies. Nine of the studies (77.8%) showed that the prognosis, infection and mortality rate of COVID-19 patients was associated with vitamin D status. The majority of the published studies reviewed concluded that a COVID-19 patients vitamin D status (blood levels) can be used to determine the seriousness of COVID-

19, risk of being infected with COVID-19, and death from COVID-19. Hence, maintaining appropriate levels of Vitamin D is recommended to cope with the pandemic.

Vitamin D Synergizes with Vaccines
A 2019 study showed that taking vitamin D and then getting an influenza vaccine enhanced the levels of TGF-β in the plasma (*an immune system booster*) (*Goncalves-Mendes et al., 2019*). In another study by Patel et al., (*2019*), it was shown that taking both Vitamin D and A increased immunity, when taken with influenza vaccine in pediatric patients.

Vitamin D Reduces Admissions to ICU
In a randomized pilot study that looked at the effects of calcifediol treatment and mortality with patients hospitalized for COVID-19, found that the giving the patients high doses of calcifediol or 25-hydroxyvitamin D (25[OH]D), (the main metabolite of vitamin D) reduced significantly the need for ICU care in patients hospitalized with COVID-19 [9].

Geographical Latitude and COVID-19 Cases
A fourfold association was discovered among people diagnosed with COVID-19, latitude and vitamin D deficiency. The sole cause of this is because D is made in the body with the help of sunshine. Hence many European countries receive little sunlight through the year due to their geographical latitude [10].

In another study looking at 20 European countries a significant correlation was found between vitamin D levels and COVID-19 cases [11].

Sunlight Kills Bad Bacteria

Studies have shown that the ultra-violet and infra-red radiation present in sunlight act as natural virucidal elements, which kill bad viruses and bacteria (*Lytle and Sagripanti, 2005; Martin et al., 2009*).

Engineered Good Bacteria to help defeat COVID-19
Ivermectin

Ivermectin is a substance that comes from a certain bacteria. However it has some lethal effects. These ill-effects can be removed by chemically re-designing the compound. Ivermectin has been shown to impede various parasitic infections, including certain cancers. A recent study discovered Ivermectin was effective in destroying COVID-19 incidence in cell cultures (*Caly et al., 2020*).

Studies confirm COVID-19 Patients have Low Levels of Vitamin D

Adults admitted to Inha University Hospital in South Korea discovered extreme vitamin D deficiency in 24% of their COVID-19 patients, compared to 7.3% in the control group [12].

Also a 2020 study by Mendy and colleagues discovered that COVID-19 patients were more likely to be deficient in vitamin D compared to people without COVID-19 [13].

In Israel a study found low vitamin D levels were associated with a higher likelihood of contracting COVID-19 [14].

Another study looking at COVID-19 in patients who were suffering from Parkinson's disease in Lombardy, Italy discovered their patients were less likely to have received vitamin D supplementation compared to patients who were uninfected [15].

Further Reading
Effects of Vitamin D on COVID-19 Infection and Prognosis: A Systematic Review. Hiwot Yisak et al. 2021.

Coconut Oil
Researchers highlighted preliminary research on the antiviral effects of lauric acid, which is found in coconut oil and its metabolite, monolaurin. They stated that a clinical trial involved participants consuming 3 tablespoons of virgin coconut oil daily along with 800 mg of monolaurin in patients suffering from COVID-19 helped improve their recovery [15a].

Omega 3's Help Fight COVID-19
Omega-3s are also called in the scientific literature "n-3s". They exist in flaxseed, flaxseed oil and fish. High levels of DHA in the body are found in the body's brain, retina (eye) and sperm cells. These are all regions that store high amounts of membrane electrical energy. A recent research study concluded that Omega-3 fatty acids, with special emphasis on docosahexaenoic acid (DHA) and eicosapentaenoic acid (EPA) exhibit anti-inflammatory effects that may reduce some COVID-19 patients' need for intensive care. The study further states that Omega-3 fatty acids supplementation in order to help fight COVID-19 cannot be fully recommended until controlled and randomized trials are carried out [16].

COVID-19 Herbal Sachets
Besides sunlight being able to kill bad viruses, herbal sachets may also help. The government of Heilongjiang in China has suggested a herbal sachet to be carried on one's person in order to help ward off the COVID-19 virus. The scented sachet designed to repel the influenza virus as well

as other viruses is composed of Cinnamomum camphora, Realgar, Angelica dahurica, Artemisia argyi and Pogostemon cablin, Eupatorium fortune. The report also states that herbs decocted to fumigate the body include – Acorus tatarinowii, Valerianajatamansi Jones, Perilla frutescens, Artemisia argyi and Mentha haplocalyx. Overall the herbs in the sachet are designed to strengthen the body's resistance to viruses and remove dampness [17].

Numbered References. Chapter 2

(1) Inhibition of NF-B-Mediated Inflammation in Severe Acute Respiratory Syndrome Coronavirus Infected Mice Increases Survival. DeDiego, M.L et al. J. Virol. 2014, 88, 913-924.

(2) Natural small molecules as inhibitors of coronavirus lipid-dependent attachment to host cells: A possible strategy for reducing SARS-COV-2 infectivity? Baglivo, M et al. Vergoten, G. Glycyrrhizin: An alternative drug for the treatment of COVID-19 infection and the associated res-piratory syndrome? Pharmacol. Ther. 2020, 214, 107618.

(2a) Propolis, Bee Honey, and Their Components Protect against Coronavirus Disease 2019 (COVID-19): A Review of In Silico. Amira Mohammed Ali et al. Feb 2021.

(3) Antiviral activity of dried extract of Stevia. Kedik, S.A. et al. Pharm. Chem. J. 2009, 43, 198-199.

(4) Vitamin D sufficiency, a serum 25-hydroxyvitamin D at least 30 ng/mL reduced risk for adverse clinical outcomes in patients with COVID-19 infection. Zhila Maghbooli et al. Sept 2020.

(5) P. Mehta, D. F. Mcauley, M. Brown, E. Sanchez, R. S. Tattersall, and J. J. Manson, "COVID-19: consider cytokine storm syndromes and immunosuppression," The Lancet, vol. 395, no. 10229, pp. 1033-1034, 2020.

(6) Traditional Chinese herbal medicine at the forefront battle against COVID19: Clinical experience and scientific basis. David Y.W. Lee et al. Sept 2020.

(7) Abu-Mouch et al., 2011) and HCV genotype 2-3 (Nimer and Mouch, 2012.

(8) Herbal immune-boosters: Substantial warriors of pandemic Covid-19 battle. Kanika Khannaa et al. Sept 2020.

(9) Entrenas Castillo M, Entrenas Costa LM, Vaquero Barrios JM, et al. Effect of calcifediol treatment and best available therapy versus best available therapy on intensive care unit admission and mortality among patients hospitalized for COVID-19: a pilot randomized clinical study. J Steroid Biochem Mol Biol. 2020;203:105751. doi:10. 1016/j.jsbmb.2020.105751.

(10) Kara M, Ekiz T, Ricci V, Kara Ö. 'Scientific strabismus' or two related pandemics: COVID-19 & vitamin D deficiency. Br J Nutr. 2020;1-20.

(11) Ali N. Role of vitamin D in preventing of COVID-19 infection, progression and severity. J Infect Public Health. 2020;13(10):1373-1380. doi:10.1016/j.jiph.2020.06.021.

(12) Im JH, Je YS, Baek J, Chung M-H, Kwon HY, Lee J-S. Nutritional status of patients with coronavirus disease 2019 (COVID-19). Int J Infect Dis. 2020;100:390-393. doi:10.1016/j.ijid.2020.08.018.

(13) Mendy A, Apewokin S, Wells AA, Morrow AL. Factors associated with hospitalization and disease severity in a racially and ethnically diverse population of COVID-19 patients.

(14) Merzon E, Tworowski D, Gorohovski A, et al. Low plasma 25 (OH) vitamin D level is associated with increased risk of COVID-19 infection: an Israeli population-based study. FEBS J. 2020;287 (17):3693-3702. doi:10.1111/febs.15495.

(15) Fasano A, Cereda E, Barichella M, et al. COVID 19 in parkinson's disease patients living in Lombardy, Italy. Mov Disorders. 2020;35 (7):1089-1093. doi:10.1002/mds.28176.

(15a) The Potential of Coconut Oil and its Derivatives as Effective and Safe Antiviral Agents Against the Novel Coronavirus (nCoV-2019).

(16) Potential benefits and risks of omega-3 fatty acids supplementation to patients with COVID-19
Marcelo M. Rogero. et al. July 2020.

(17) M.Y. Zhong, Q. Liu, L.M. Zhang, D.M. Lu, Y. Chen, J. Qing, The application of influenza scents in the prevention of COVID-19, China's Naturopathy. 28 (11) (2020) 1-3.

Chapter 3. Exploring DCA, EPA and Omega 3's for the Prevention of COVID-19.

While on the topic of prevention of COVID-19, I would like to point out a study involving Lactoferrin. I first came across Lactoferrin in my anti-aging research years ago. Lactoferrin is a naturally occurring glycoprotein that is non-toxic, found in dairy and is easily obtained as a nutritional supplement. In a recent study titled: *Lactoferrin as potential preventative and adjunct treatment for COVID-19* that was conducted by Raymond Chang and colleagues and published in September 2020, the authors stated that Lactoferrin exhibited antiviral efficacy (in vitro) against a wide variety of viruses, including SARS-CoV, which is a coronavirus closely related to SARS-CoV-2. The authors concluded that Lactoferrn exhibits unique anti-inflammatory effects that may be relevant to severe COVID-19 cases.

Fish Oil Contains DHA and EPA
DHA and EPA are present in fish because they become synthesized by the microalgae and not directly by the fish themselves. Hence as a fish consumes phytoplankton that has consumed microalgae, the fish build-up omega-3s in their bodily tissues.

A 2019 study conducted by Gerling and colleagues showed that young men given fish oil (3g EPA + 2g DHA/day) for 3 months exhibited increases levels of DHA and EPA in their muscles as well as in their mitochondrial membranes [1]. According to the USDA National Nutrient Database (*Release 28. Nutrients: 20:5 n-3 (EPA)*), EPA can be found in abundance in Menhaden Fish oil, Herring, Salmon and   Sardines.

Further Reading
Bistrian B.R. Parenteral fish oil emulsions in critically ill COVID-19 emulsions. J. Parenter. Enteral Nutr. 2020 doi: 10.1002/jpen.1871.

Stapleton R.D., Martin J.M., Mayer K. Fish oil in critical illness: mechanisms and clinical applications. Crit. Care Clin. 2010;26:501–514. doi: 10.1016/j.ccc.2010.04.009.

Mancuso P., Whelan J., DeMichele S.J., Snider C.C., Guszcza J.A., Karlstad M.D. Dietary fish oil and fish and borage oil suppress intrapulmonary proinflammatory eicosanoid biosynthesis and attenuate pulmonary neutrophil accumulation in endotoxic rats. Crit. Care Med. 1997;25:1198–1206.

How Much DHA and EPA does my body require?
The recommended daily allowance for DHA and EPA is 1 gram per day; preferably from oily fish. Supplements can also be used [2]. This may not seem like a large amount, but it is the ability for these acids to be easily absorbed into the body that gives them their effectiveness.

Where can I find Docosahexaenoic and Eicosapentaenoic acids?
Fish are one source, however choose fish that are low in mercury. Examples include herring, salmon, sardines, and trout. DHA and EPA can also be obtained from krill oil and fish oil [3].

How DHA is made in the body from ALA

When you eat foods that are abundant in ALA (alpha-linolenic acid) your body converts the ALA into EPA, which is then converted to DHA. This conversion takes place in your liver with a conversion rate of approximately 15% [4]. ALA is found in abundance in Flaxseed Oil (linseed), Canola oils and Soybeans with moderate amounts in Walnut and Chia Seeds [5] [6].

EPA and DHA in Fish

The highest levels of EPA and DHA are found in 3 ounces of Salmon, Atlantic (wild, cooked), followed by Sardines in tomato sauce, followed by 3 ounces of cooked rainbow Trout [7] [8].

Where do I Obtain Omega-3s?

Certain brands of yogurt, juices, eggs, milk and soy are fortified with DHA and other omega-3s [9].

Since the year 2002 food manufacturers begun adding DHA and arachidonic acid to most infant formulas in the United States. Beef is low in omega-3s. However, beef from grass-fed cows contains higher levels of omega-3s.

Omega-3s can also be obtained from cod liver oil, fish oil, krill oil and vegetarian products that contain algal oil. A standard fish oil has approximately 1,000 mg of fish oil, which is made up of 180 mg EPA and 120 mg DHA. However doses can vary widely [10].

Cod liver oil supplements also contain vitamin D and vitamin A in addition to LC omega-3s. Krill oil has omega-3s primarily in the form of phospholipids. Research also suggests these are more bioavailable by the body than the standard omega-3s found in fish oil [11].

Vegetarian Sources of Omega 3's
Algal oil provides approximately 100 to 300 mg of DHA, with some brands containing EPA. The supplement forms also include omega-3s in the triglyceride form (12).

According to a research study, the bioavailability of DHA from algal oil was found to be equivalent to that of cooked salmon [13].

What types of Fish are abundant in Omega 3's?
The omega-3 contents in fish have a wide variation. Cold-water fatty fish, such as tuna, herring, salmon, mackerel and sardines contain an abundance of omega-3s [14]. Farmed fish contain higher amounts of DHA and EPA compared to wild-caught fish, depending upon what the farmed fish have been fed [15] [16]. For example, farm-raised Atlantic salmon from Scotland showed a decrease in their DHA and EPA levels between 2006 and 2015. This decline was due to a change in the marine ingredients that were present in the fish feed [17].

Signs of Low Omega 3's in the body
If a person lacks healthy levels of essential fatty acids (omega-3s or omega-6s) their skin will be more rough, scaly and one may be more prone to dermatitis [18].

Closing Summary
Populations living in regions where fish are plentiful will fare better during the COVID-19 pandemic. As a matter of fact, according to research done by John Hopkins, countries with the lowest COVID-19 deaths (as of November 2020) Papua New Guinea, Iceland, New Zealand and Vietnam are regions where the majority of the population resides along the coast. However in undeveloped countries the mercury in fish may present a problem [19]. Tuna consumption should be limited (a maximum of 6oz per week) due to mercury.

Also high levels of methyl mercury have been found in Kingfish, Swordfish, Mackerel, Shark and Tilefish [20]. High levels of metyl mercury have also been found in Pacific oysters and some trout [21]. However fish raised in fish farms in water that is free of mercury may experience a boom in demand in the future.

Why the Demand for Acerola juice will soar in the coming years
From my research I have discovered that the juice highest in both EPA and DHA is Acerola juice. Acerola juice happens to be one of the foods highest in Vitamin C.

Foods highest in Vitamin C
According to the USDA National Nutrient Database
the top 3 foods abundant in Vitamin C are Acerola juice, raw, followed by Acerola, (west indian cherry), and Rose Hips, wild (Northern Plains Indians) with Oranges ranking 4th [22].

DHA Levels in Drinks
According to the USDA National Nutrient Database, drinks most abundant in DHA are Acerola juice, daiquiri and 100 proof gin, rum, vodka and whiskey) [23].

According to the USDA National Nutrient Database Liquids that contain the highest levels of EPA are found in -
Acerola juice, Beer, daiquiri and 100 proof gin, rum, vodka and whiskey [24].

In short summary, besides a possible increase / shortage of Acerola juice, we may also witness an increase in beer, daiquiri and 100 proof gin, rum, vodka and whiskey consumption as the pandemic continues to sweep the globe.

Vitamin C helps people Diagnosed with COVID-19

An in-depth meta-analysis study looking at vitamin C in treating and preventing the common cold was carried out by Hemil¨ a and Chalker (*2013*). The study concluded that vitamin C mega dosing reduced the frequency of the common cold throughout the community. An above average intake of Vitamin C may help people who are critically ill with COVID-19. A review of several studies found a daily dose of 1,000 to 6,000 mg of vitamin C taken either by mouth or intravenously shortened the time on ventilation by about 25% (*Hemila J Intens Care 2020*).

Numbered References. Chapter 3

(1) Gerling C.J., Mukai K., Chabowski A., Heigenhauser G.J.F., Holloway G.P., Spriet L.L., Jannas-Vela S. Incorporation of omega-3 fatty acids into human skeletal muscle sarcolemmal and mitochondrial membranes following 12 weeks of fish oil supplementation. Front. Physiol. 2019;10:348. doi: 10.3389/fphys.2019.00348.

(2) Omega-3 Fatty Acids. Fact Sheet for Health Professionals. www.NIH.gov.

(3) Omega-3 Fatty Acids. Fact Sheet for Health Professionals. www.NIH.gov.

(4) Harris WS. Omega-3 fatty acids. In: Coates PM, Betz JM, Blackman MR, et al., eds. Encyclopedia of Dietary Supplements. 2nd ed. London and New York: Informa Healthcare; 2010:577-86.

(5) Jones PJH, Papamandjaris AA. Lipids: cellular metabolism. In: Erdman JW, Macdonald IA, Zeisel SH, eds. Present Knowledge in Nutrition. 10th ed. Washington, DC: Wiley-Blackwell; 2012:132-48.

(6) Harris WS. Omega-3 fatty acids. In: Coates PM, Betz JM, Blackman MR, et al., eds. Encyclopedia of Dietary Supplements. 2nd ed. London and New York: Informa Healthcare; 2010:577-86

(7) USDA National Nutrient Database for Standard Reference. Release 28. Nutrients: 20:5 n-3 (EPA) (g)

(8) USDA National Nutrient Database for Standard Reference. Release 28. Nutrients: 22:6 n-3 (DHA) (g)

(9) U.S. Food and Drug Administration. Questions & answers for consumers concerning infant formula.

(10) National Institutes of Health. Dietary Supplement Label Database.external link disclaimer 2015.

(11) ConsumerLab.com. Product review: fish oil and omega-3 fatty acid supplements review (including krill, algae, calamari, green-lipped mussel oil).

(12) ConsumerLab.com. Product review: fish oil and omega-3 fatty acid supplements review (including krill, algae, calamari, green-lipped mussel oil).

(13) Arterburn LM, Oken HA, Bailey Hall E, Hamersley J, Kuratko CN, Hoffman JP. Algal-oil capsules and cooked salmon: nutritionally equivalent sources of docosahexaenoic acid. J Am Diet Assoc 2008;108:1204-9.

(14) Harris WS. Omega-3 fatty acids. In: Coates PM, Betz JM, Blackman MR, et al., eds. Encyclopedia of Dietary Supplements. 2nd ed. London and New York: Informa Healthcare; 2010:577-86.

(15) Miller MR, Nichols PD, Carter CG. n-3 Oil sources for use in aquaculture-alternatives to the unsustainable harvest of wild fish. Nutr Res Rev 2008;21:85-96.

(16) Cladis DP, Kleiner AC, Freiser HH, Santerre CR. Fatty acid profiles of commercially available finfish fillets in the United States. Lipids 2014;49:1005-18.

(17) Sprague M, Dick JR, Tocher DR. Impact of sustainable feeds on omega-3 long-chain fatty acid levels in farmed Atlantic salmon, 2006-2015. Sci Rep 2016;6:21892.

(18) Institute of Medicine, Food and Nutrition Board. Dietary reference intakes for energy, carbohydrate, fiber, fat, fatty acids, cholesterol, protein, and amino acids (macronutrients). Washington, DC: National Academy Press; 2005.

(19) U.S. Food and Drug Administration. Fish: what pregnant women and parents should know.external link disclaimer 2014.

(20) U.S. Food and Drug Administration. Fish: what pregnant women and parents should know.external link disclaimer 2014.

(21) Omega-3 Fatty Acids. Fact Sheet for Health Professionals (www.mih.giv).

(22) USDA National Nutrient Database for Standard Reference. Release 28. Nutrients: Vitamin C, total ascorbic acid (mg).

(23) USDA National Nutrient Database for Standard Reference. Release 28. Nutrients: 22:6 n-3 (DHA) (g).

(24) USDA National Nutrient Database for Standard Reference. Release 28. Nutrients: 20:5 n-3 (EPA) (g).

Chapter 4. How Edhedra is being used for the Prevention and Treatment of COVID-19.

Before moving onto Ephedra Herbs I would like to first bring to light a herb used in India called Ashwagandha. Ashwagandha contains an abundance of Withanone (*Ran Gao et al. Sept 2014*) which is why it has been scientifically proven to kill cancer cells [1]. In a research study titled: *Withanone from Withania somnifera Attenuates SARS-CoV-2 RBD and Host ACE2 Interactions to Rescue Spike Protein Induced Pathologies in Humanized Zebrafish Model* that was conducted by Acharya Balkrishna and colleagues and published in March 2021 found that withanone and withaferin A, which are phytochemicals in Withania somnifera exhibit substances that inhibit the entry of viruses into cells. An extract of Withanone from W. somnifera was tested for its ability to reduce the infection of SARS-CoV-2 into cells in humanized zebrafish. The study found that Withanone prepared from W. somnifera leaves stopped human-like pathological responses induced in humanized zebrafish by SARS-CoV-2 recombinant spike (S) protein. The study concluded that withanone acts as a very potent inhibitor of SARS-CoV-2 coronavirus entry into host cells.

Ephedra for Treatment and Prevention of COVID-19
Ephedra used alone is very dangerous, which is why it has been banned in some countries. To date, Ephedra is currently banned for sale in the United States of America. The best way to use ephedra is to combine it in small amounts with the appropriate herbs. This is because ephedra assists the healing properties of herbs, acting as a

kind of healing synergist. This means it can greatly enhance the healing effects of specific herbal formulas. Let's look at the scientific evidence to see why this is so.

Two recent reviews on Traditional Chinese Herbal Medicine illustrate how TCM may be of use in helping defeat COVID-19. In the first review, the authors state a herbal formula that was used in the H1N1 outbreak that may be useful for preventing COVID-19 (*Luo et al., 2020*). The second review states guidelines for the treatment of COVID-19; using various stages (*Ang et al., 2020a*). The most cited herb was Ephedra. Ephedra is used for treating asthma, cough, cold and for losing weight.

Ephedra methyl. Ephedrine contains pseudoephedrine D and L-ephedrine which exhibits anti-influenza virus activity. This occurs due to its ability to inhibit the pathways responsible for viral replication and by modulating inflammatory reactions and adjusting host Toll-like receptors (*TLRs; Zhang et al., 2019*) and inducing gene protein (RIG-I) (via retinoic acid) (*Wei et al., 2019*).

Ephedrine has been shown to inhibit the infection of canine renal cells caused by the H1N1 influenza virus via a concentration-dependent manner (*Hyuga et al., 2016*). The tannic acid of Ephedra sinensis extract has been shown to inhibit acidification of lysosomes and endosomes in a dose-dependent manner. In turn this was shown to inhibit the growth of the influenza A infection in canine renal cells (*Mantani et al., 1999*).

Ephedra contains the alkaloid ephedrine, whose serious side effects affect the cardiovascular and nervous system, resulting in some deaths (*FDA, 2008; EFSA, 2013; EMA, 2015b*). Hence, if it must be used, it must be done so with great care and preferably under a doctor's supervision.

The Amygdalus Communis Vas Formula
A study examining the herbs Ephedra and Amygdalus researched if they had high potential for treating COVID-19 [1a]. The study found that combining Amygdalus with Ephedra exhibited a high confidence scale making it potentially useful for treating all stages of COVID-19. The study goes on to state that 44 potential targets and 26 active ingredients may reduce COVID-19 infections. The main ingredients in Amygdalus were found to be quercetin, luteolin, kaempferol which target Interleukin 6 (IL-6) and NF-kB. The study concluded that combining Amygdalus with Ephedra may have therapeutic effects against COVID-19. The method of action was by affecting pathological processes such as immune responses, inflammatory responses, cell apoptosis, hypoxia damage as well as other pathological processes via multiple components.

Ephedra Helps Lower Cytokine Storms. The Maxing Ganshi decoction
The Maxing Ganshi decoction is made of Ephedra sinica Stapf (ephedra), Glycyrrhiza uralensis Fisch. (licorice root), Semen Armeniacae Amarum (almonds) and Gypsum (gypsum). The active ingredients are - quercetin, kaempferol, delphinidin, herbacetin and resivit. The Quercetin and kaempferol may inhibit coagulation pathways triggered by IL-6. It may also help reduce cytokine storms [2].

Ephedra for Inhibiting Influenza and Pneumonia
Yinhuapinggan granule (YHPG) is a medicine granule containing Ephedra [3]. It is based upon Ma-Huang-Tang (Ephedra Decoction) as well as from the clinical experiences of Professor Wan Haitong. This formula was shown to inhibit the growth of the influenza virus (in vitro).

Ephedra-bitter almonds
Ephedra-bitter almonds have been used to prevent as well as treat COVID-19 by inhibiting the virus directly. This in turn expressed a healthy response upon the immune system [4].

A research paper titled: *Diagnosis and Treatment Protocol for Novel Coronavirus Pneumonia* that was published by the National Health Commission & State Administration of Traditional Chinese Medicine on March 3, 2020 states that for severe COVID cases the following lung-strengthening and poison purging formula is recommended. It is used when the symptoms of fever, flushing, yellowish phlegm, or blood in sputum, tiredness, nausea, cough, wheezing, shortness of breath, food loss, fatigue, poor stool and short urination or dryness and stickiness are present in the patient. The formula is listed as -

Raw ephedra 6g, fragrant fragrant 10g (back), almond 9g, raw gypsum 15g, licorice 3g, Magnolia 10g, atractylodes 15g, grass fruit, gardenia 10g, 10g, pinellia 9g, Poria 15g, raw rhubarb 5g (back) 10g and red peony 10g.

Preparation and Dosages
Herbs are boiled in 100 to 200ml of water. Taken once or twice daily.

The same research paper states that for mild COVID cases that this formula relieves cold dampness and stagnation lung syndrome. It is used in patients that display the following symptoms: nausea, fatigue, sore body, cough, expectoration, chest tightness, fever, appetite, suffocation, loss of vomiting and sticky stools. The formula is made up of the following herbs -

Raw ephedra 6g, raw gypsum 15g, almond 9g, loquat 15g, gardenia 15g, Peilan 9g, Cangzhu 15g, Yunling 45g, Atractylodes 30g, Guanzhong 9g, Dilong 15g, Xu Changqing 15g, Huoxiang 15g, Jiao Sanxian 9g each, yarrow fruit 9g, Magnolia officinalis 15g, betel coconut 9g and ginger 15g.

Preparation and Dosages
Herbs are Boiled in 600ml water. This is than drank three times a day; at morning, noon and evening before meals.

Further Reading
Screening of antiviral components of Ma Huang Tang and investigation on the Ephedra alkaloids efficacy on influenza virus type a. Wei W, Du H, Shao C, Zhou H, Lu Y, Yu L, et al. Front Pharmacol. 2019;10:961. doi: 10.3389/fphar.2019.00961.

Combining Ephedra with Glycyrrhiza
When Ephedra is combined with Glycyrrhiza it exhibits powerful healing effects. This combination is frequently prescribed to treat COVID-19. A research study hypothesized that the Ephedra-Glycyrrhiza drug pair is a potential choice for the treatment of COVID-19. 112 active compounds were identified from the Ephedra combo Glycyrrhiza via a network pharmacology approach [5]. The Ephedra-Glycyrrhiza pair analysis showed these compounds may positively affect the body's respiratory, blood circulation, nervous system and digestive systems; offering organ protection, antiviral benefits and immune regulation. Simulations involving molecular docking showed the active compounds in the Ephedra Glycyrrhiza combo bound well to COVID-19 related targets, including the protease Mpro (also called 3CLpro) as well as the spike protein and ACE2. The study concluded that the Ephedra-Glycyrrhiza combo be further explored for the treatment of

COVID-19 via its ability to act through multiple targets and pathways.

Glycyrrhiza in Detail
Glycyrrhizin is the major bioactive component of Glycyrrhiza. This has been scientifically confirmed to interact directly with ACE2. Hence it is suggested that glycyrrhizin may act as a therapeutic agent against patients being treated for COVID-19 (*Zhou et al., 2020*).

What does ACE2 mean?
ACE2 is short for angiotensin-converting enzyme 2 (ACE2). It acts as the main host cell receptor of human pathogenic coronaviruses. In theory, herbs that down-regulate ACE2 may provide a starting defense against viral infections. During the SARS outbreak, Taiwanese researchers stated emodin was an inhibitor of both S and ACE2 proteins. Emodin can be found in Polygonum multiflorum Thunb and Rheum officinale Baill (*Ho et al., 2007*). Other herbs identified as potential enhancers of ACE2 expression, include curcumin, rosmarinic acid, baicalin, tanshinones and magnolol (*ANSES, 2020*).

Ephedrine reduces coughing
An extract of ephedrine (at a dose of 200 mg/kg) was shown to reduce coughing up to 68.3% [6].

Ephedra relieves Asthma
When Ephedrae was combined with Armeniacae Semen (in 2:1 ratio) it exhibited better therapeutic effects on relieving asthma and coughing than similar combinations. This significant reduction may be due to the down-regulation of CGRP level and a variety of inflammatory cytokines [7].

The Huashi baidu Granule Formula
This formula was used in Jinyintan Hospital on a total of 146 cases. 109 patients were completely cured of COVID-19 and discharged using this formula (a discharge rate of 74.7%). The Huashibaidu Granule Formula was also given to 124 moderate COVID cases in Dongxihu Fangcang Hospital, China as well as 894 mild to moderate COVID-19 cases [8] [9]. No adverse events or kidney or liver damage was reported in any of the patients who received this formula.

The Huashi Baidu formula (HSBD) consists of Ephedra sinica Stapf, Glycyrrhiza glabra L, Agastache rugosa (Fisch.&C.A.Mey) and Gypsum Magnolia officinalis Rehder&E.H.Wilson, Atractylodes lancea (Thunb.) DC, Prunus armeniaca L, Gypsum Fibrosum, Astragalus mongholicus Bunge, Eruca sativa Mill, Radix Paeoniae Rubra, which is added or subtracted from MXSGD, HXZQ powders, Amomum tsaoko Crevost et Lemarie, Pinellia pedatisecta Schott, Poria cocos (Schw.)Wolf, Rheum officinale Bail and Xuanbai Chengqi decoction [8] [9].

Numbered References. Chapter 4

Withanone-Rich Combination of Ashwagandha Withanolides. Restricts Metastasis and Angiogenesis through hnRNP-K. Ran Gao et al. Sept 2014.

(1a) The Important Herbal Pair for the Treatment of COVID-19 and Its Possible Mechanisms. Shujie Xia et al. Fujian University of Traditional Chinese Medicine.

(2) Immunotherapeutic implications of IL-6 blockade for cytokine storm. Tanaka, M. Narazaki et al. Immunotherapy, 8 (8) (2016), pp. 959-970.

(3) Protective effects of Yinhuapinggan granule on mice with influenza viral pneumonia.Xue-qianPeng et al Jan 2006.

(4) Exploring active ingredients and function mechanisms of Ephedra-bitter almond for prevention and treatment of Corona virus disease 2019 (COVID-19) based on network pharmacology.

(5) Chemical composition and pharmacological mechanism of ephedra-glycyrrhiza drug pair against coronavirus disease 2019 (COVID-19). Xiaoling Li et al.

(6) Manno K, Yamamoto S, Suga A, Kurio W. Antitussive effect of crude drugs contained preparation (Asgen®): combined effects on the cough reflex induced by electrical stimulation in Guinea pigs. Pharmacometrics. 1993;46:211-6.

(7) Liu X, Yang Z. Study on antitussive and antiasthmatic effects of different compatibility ratio of ephedra and almond. Clin Res Pract. 2019;4:8-9.

(8) Research progress of traditional Chinese medicine against COVID-19. Wei Ren et al. February 2021.

(9) X.W. Yang, Material basis research of Anti-COVID-19 Huashibaidu granule gormula, Modern Chinese medicine 22 (5) (2020) 672-689.

Chapter 5. Chinese Herbs Scientifically Proven to Treat and Prevent COVID-19.

Next I want to share with the reader the very best Chinese herbs scientifically proven to treat and prevent COVID-19. Some of these herbal formulas have shown remarkable success. For example, The Qingfei paidu Decoction has shown an overall relief rate of COVID-19 symptoms of 93% (*Liu et al., 2020a*) and The Qingfei Paidu decoction, used to treat 214 confirmed cases of COVID-19, exhibited an effective treatment rate of up to 92% (*Zhao et al., 2020*) [1].
As of March 2021, Qingfei Paidu decoction (QFPDD) has been approved as a general prescription for treatment of COVID-19 in China (*Wei Ren et al. Feb 2021*).

Traditional Chinese Medicines (TCM) for treating COVID-19. Throughout China's history, it is estimated that over 100 herbal TCM formulas have been exclusively developed for saving people's lives during pandemics (*David Y.W. Lee et al. Sept 2020*). TCM is now credited for the successful battle against COVID-19 patients in China (*Lu and Lu, 2020*). This may be the sole reason why China, with the world's largest population does not have as many deaths from COVID-19 as in the United States or Brazil.

COVID-19 Symptomology
COVID-19 symptoms are similar to those outlined in the plague category of Huang Di Nei Jing (Inner Canon of the Yellow Emperor) for being highly infectious and epidemic. COVID-19 symptoms are also similar to those discussed in Shang Han Za Bing Lun (Treatise on Febrile and

Miscellaneous Diseases) which was authored by Zhongjing Zhang. The Treatise divides epidemic symptoms into warm (A type of disease that exhibits main symptom of fever that is caused by warm pathogen) as well as cold (This is a disease type that exhibits symptoms of exogenous fever that is caused by cold pathogens). Hence, because the majority of COVID-19 cases exhibit symptoms of body aches, fear of cold and fatigue, COVID-19 belongs to the category of typhoid virus and should be dialectical as typhoid fever. Hence, a few prescriptions in Treatise on Febrile and Miscellaneous Diseases exist. These include The Maxing Shigan decoction, The Qingfei Paidu decoction, The Shegan Mahuang decoction and The Xiaochaihu decoction. These are already in popular use in mainland China for removing symptoms of cold pathogens [1a] [1b]. Now let's move onto Chinese herbs proven to defeat COVID-19.

Herbal formulas used for treating severe COVID-19 patients

The Maxinshigan Tang Formula [1c]
Yang et al. performed LC-MS/MS and integrated network analysis to identify the active components of Ma-Xin-Shi-Gan and their possible mechanism of action (*Yang et al., 2020*). The researchers discovered flavonoids, glycosides, carboxylic acids and saponins. Glycyrrhizic acid in particular, isolated from Ma-Xin-Shi-Gan, exerted anti-inflammatory effects by blocking toll-like-receptors as well as suppressing IL-6 production in macrophage. Huang et al. discovered that quercetin, luteolin, isorhamnetin, baicalein, naringenin, kaempferol and wogonin were the main active compounds responsible for its potency (*Huang et al., 2020*).

These herbs are boiled together in 1000ml of pure water for 30 minutes; after boiling to get a 600ml tincture. Each tincture is than subdivided into three doses. These are drank in 200ml portions three times daily. The formula is as follows -

Ephedra 15g
Licorice 9g
Almond 10g
Plaster 20g

The Baihegujin Tang Formula
This formula is a great alternative if you do not have access to Ephedra. This formula is also for treating severe COVID-19 cases [1d].

Licorice 3g	Ophiopogon 6g
Dihuang 15g	Angelica 15g
Shudihuang 15g	White peony 6g
Xuanshen 10g	Lily 6g
Chinese bellflower 6g	Beimu 6g

These herbs are also boiled together in 1000ml of pure water for 30 minutes; after boiling to get a 600ml tincture. Each tincture is than subdivided into three doses. These are drank in 200ml portions three times daily.

The Lian-Hua-Qing-Wen Formula
A study by Li et al. researched the potency of Lian-Hua-Qing-Wen. Lian-Hua-Qing-Wen is a commercialized herbal formulation designed to specifically inhibit SARS-CoV-2 infection of Vero E6 cells (*Runfeng et al., 2020*). The study found Lian-Hua-Qing-Wen significantly inhibited SARS-CoV-2 replication in Vero E6 cells as well as reduced pro-inflammatory cytokines. Although its IC50 at over 400 µg/ml is a far cry from the efficiency of remdesivir this research

study shows that this herbal formula can be validated as an ideal prophylactic considering its very mild toxicity.

The next group of herbs I am next about to share with the reader in this chapter come from a recent published study that was produced in association with McLean Hospital/Harvard Medical School, Henan University of Chinese Medicine and the Institute of Pharmaceutical and Biomedical Sciences at Johannes Gutenberg University in Germany. The published study is titled: *Traditional Chinese herbal medicine at the forefront battle against COVID19: Clinical experience and scientific basis (David Y.W. Lee et al. Sept 2020)*.

Glycyrrhiza glabra L. - Fabaceae (Roots) Many of these herbs used to successfully treat and prevent COVID-19 contain the substance Glycyrrhizin. Glycyrrhizin found in Glycyrrhiza glabra root (licorice herb) is abundant in flavonoids, glycyrrhetinic acid, β- a sitosterol, hydroxyl coumarins β-sitosterol and hydroxyl coumarins. Glycyrrhiza is used for coughs and / or sore throat (*WHO, 1999; EMA, 2012a*).

Glycyrrhiza has been shown to impede the viral replication of SARS-CoV (*Nourazarian et al., 2016; Keyaerts et al., 2007*). This unique plant would make for a great trial drug in COVID-19 affected patients; possibly developing it as a potent cure drug (*Chen et al., 2004; Cinatl et al., 2003; Brush et al., 2006*). Glycyrrhizin has been shown to exhibit anti-inflammatory inflammation effects (*Ramos-Tovar et al., 2020*).

Additional studies confirm that Glycyrrhizin inhibited both virus replication and SARS-CoV in cells. A 2003 report [2] examining the effects of glycyrrhizin in several stages of infection of Vero cells reported glycyrrhizin was the most effective agent (EC50 300 mg/L).

This study spurred the development of several glycyrrhizin analogues which in turn exhibited potent SARS replication inhibitory activity. The study discovered glycyrrhizin significantly decreased proinflammatory cytokines (namely IL-6, IL-8 and TNF). This suggests it reduces proinflammatory responses of host cells during viral infection [3].

What does IL-6, IL-8 mean?
IL is short for Interleukins, which are a group of related proteins that are made by the body's leukocytes (white blood cells). Interleukins regulate the body's immune responses. Interleukins can also be artificially made in labs. These are often used to boost the body's immune system in people diagnosed with cancer.

A hydroethanolic extract of Glycyrrhizin (100 mg/kg, p.o) was shown to exert antiasthma activity (similar effect to prednisolone) (10 mg/kg, p.o.) in mast cells degranulation (*Patel et al., 2017*). Glycyrrhizin has also been shown to lengthen the survival time of mice that were infected with Influenza. Glycyrrhizin also inhibited the SARS-related coronavirus proliferation in vitro. Glycyrrhizic acid was shown to inhibit inflammatory cytokines and the cytopathic effect of the Respiratory Syncytial Virus (RSV) (*Fiore et al., 2008*).

More recently, research studies conducted during 2020 revealed that Glycyrrhizin lowered the ability of SARS-Cov agents to attach to cells; particularly during the early stages of viral penetration and exhibited similar behavior against COVID-19 by acting as a potential inhibitor (*Mohammadi and Shaghaghi, 2020*). Similar observations were also made by Pilcher (*2003*), Cinatl et al. (*2003*) and Yeh et al. (*2013*).

Glycyrrhiza Chemical composition - Saponins (e.g., glycyrrhizin); triterpenes (glycyrrhetinic acid); flavonoids (liquiritin, rhamnoliquirilin and liquiritigenin); coumarins (licoarylcoumarin); essential oil (*Saxena, 2005; Öztürk et al., 2017; Frattaruolo et al., 2019; El-Saber Batiha et al., 2020a*).

Glycyrrhiza Usage Directions
Based on traditional uses - 1.5 g of roots in 150 ml, as a herbal decoction taken two times daily (*EMA, 2012a*).

Further Reading
Antiviral Activity of Glycyrrhizic Acid Derivatives against SARS-Coronavirus. Hoever, G et al. J. Med. Chem. 2005, 48, 1256-1259.

Proinflammatory reducing effects of glycyrrhizin have also been confirmed with the infection of lung epithelial cells that contained the H5N1 influenza strain [4].

A Herbal Formula Recommended for the prevention and treatment of COVID-19
This formula is stated in the study mentioned earlier at the start of this chapter. The following herbal formula is recommended for protection and / or treatment for COVID-19. The formula has been created based upon the frequency of the appearance of each medicinal herb and its corresponding pharmacological activity. The herbal formula consists of four of the top herbs. It also includes herbs that have been scientifically proven to exhibit anti-virus activity as well as reduce reducing fever, remove dampness (TCM term), expel phlegm, and eliminate coughs.

The following formula is as follows -

Bupleurum chinense (10 g)	Stephania tetrandra root (10 g)
Ramulus Cinnamomi (10 g)	Polygonum cuspidate (10 g)
Scutellaria baicalensis (10 g)	Rheum palmatum (10 g)
Glycyrrhiza (15 g)	Tangerine peel (10 g)
Atractylodes macrocephala (10 g)	Semen Armeniacae Amarum (10 g)
Rhizoma Zingiberis (10 g)	Ophiopogon japonicus root (10g)
Agastache rugosa (10 g)	

The formula is combined with chaihu guizhi decoction, the Glycyrrhiza dried ginger decoction shown in "*Treatise on Febrile and Miscellaneous Diseases nowadays*" (*Shanghan Zabing Lun*, 220 AD).

In past pandemics in China, the two formulas were used for treating exogenous diseases caused by cold pathogenic factors. Currently these formulas are being used during the COVID-19 outbreak, as it conforms to the characteristics of an exogenous disease.

The Characteristics of the Herbs
Scutellaria baicalensis, Bupleurum chinense, Ramulus Cinnamomi and Glycyrrhiza restore overall harmony. Atractylodes macrocephala strengthens the body's resistance and invigorates the spleen. Agastache rugosa and Rhizoma Zingiberis warm and promote diuresis, while at the same time, the Polygonum cuspidate and the Four Stamen Stephania root have the effect of eliminating dampness. Semen Armeniacae Amarum and Tangerine peel relieve cough and lung symptoms. Polygonum cuspidate and Rheum palmatum have shown significant antiviral effects due to their rich emodin content.

Polygonum cuspidate in detail
Emodin (*found in abundance in Aloe Vera*) as well as other anthraquinone compounds in Polygonum cuspidate have been confirmed to exhibit antiviral effects. Emodin is a known anthraquinone. This has prompted studies for possible anti-HCoV activity. Emodin has also been studied for its ability to fight viral infections, although no major studies yet exist of specific cell-based direct anti-SARS-CoV activity against a real SARS strain. However Aloe emodin has been shown to bind the S protein of SARS-CoV' possibly inhibiting host cell entry [4a].

Emodin has also been shown to exhibit antiviral activity against HSV-1 and HSV-2, the parainfluenza viruses, the vaccinia virus, the pseudorabies influenza as well as others (*Sydisk et al., 1991*). Other studies have found that the bacterias Hepatitis dicoccus and Staphylococcus aureus were inhibited by emodin, emodin -8-glucoside, etc. Emodin also shows strong antibacterial activity (*Zhu et al., 1985*).

Rheum palmatum in detail
Rheum palmatum has shown major antiviral effects. It is regularly prescribed to treat certain respiratory diseases. Anthraquinone compounds that have been extracted from Rheum palmatum have been shown to inhibit the infectivity of some viruses. This in turn has been shown to inhibit the synthesis of the virus as well as its replication, and in some cases, was shown to directly inactivate the virus (*Xie et al., 2013*).

FOR PROTECTION AND PREVENTION

The following herbal formula is recommended for protection and also for treatment of COVID-19.

The Qingfei Paidu Decoction
The Qingfei Paidu Decoction consists of 21 herbs from the five classical formulae. The formula includes the herbs Ephedra sinica, Scutellaria baicalensis, Bupleurum chinense, Pogostemon cablin and Cinnamomum cassia.

A study showed that patients receiving the Qingfei Paidu decoction for three days exhibited a 84.22% rate of recovery. After six days the recovery rate was 90.15%. After nine days the recovery rate was 92.09% [4b].

A study by Yang et al. looked at the active components in the Qingfei Paidu Decoction and the Ma-Xin-Shi-Gan formula and their possible mechanism of action (*Yang et al., 2020*). The researchers discovered flavonoids, glycosides, carboxylic acids and saponins. Glycyrrhizic acid in particular, isolated from Ma-Xin-Shi-Gan, exerted anti-inflammatory effects by blocking toll-like-receptors as well as suppressing IL-6 production in macrophage. Huang et al. discovered that quercetin, luteolin, isorhamnetin, baicalein, naringenin, kaempferol and wogonin were the main active compounds responsible for its potency (*Huang et al., 2020*). [4c] Silico studies hypothesize ACE2, 3CL protein and intracellular signaling which contain COX-2, arachidonic acid, HIF-1, CASP3, MAPK, NF-κB, and Ras are potential targets of herbal medicines.

The Qingfei Paidu Decoction Effectiveness Study
Outcomes of 102 confirmed COVID-19 cases that were treated with the qingfeipaidu decoction COVID-19 symptoms were stable in 5 of the cases. In 31 cases symptoms were partially relieved in 64 cases symptoms were completely relieved. In 2 cases symptoms were aggravated. Overall the relief rate of symptoms was 93% (*Liu et al., 2020a*).

Chemical Composition of the Qingfeipaidu Decoction
A pharmacology analysis of the Qingfeipaidu Decoction (*Zhao et al., 2020*) showed the herbal formula consists of 948 various kinds of natural plant chemicals. These specific chemicals target 790 potential proteins. The interactions between this network of targets forms a highly integrated molecular network, that affects viral replication, virus invasion, and secondary forms of inflammation which are responsible for multiple organ damage in the human body with patients diagnosed with COVID-19. The Qingfeipaidu Decoction likely targets human immune related pathways and works by suppressing the activation of cytokines, as well as eliminating inflammation. Hence the formula clears the lungs and detoxes poisons from the body [4d].

FOR PROTECTION AND PREVENTION

Out of 56 prescriptions for TCM for prevention and treatment of COVID-19 in 17 hospitals in China, 79 herbs were prescribed (Wang et al., 2020). The top five herbs were as follows -

1 - Astragalus membranaceus

2 - Lonicera japonica

3 - Glycyrrhiza

4 - Atractylodes macrocephala

5 - Saposhniovia divaricata root

Lonicera japonica in detail
Lonicera japonica water extract has been shown to inhibit a wide variety of bad bacteria (Klebsiella pneumonia, cocci

and bacilli). It has also shown good inhibitory effects upon the influenza A virus (*Hu et al., 2015*). In a research study (*Zhang et al., 2019*), the authors stated that a modified lime sulfur method was used to extract the active constituents from Lonicera japonica. Also a bacteriostatic circle method was used for evaluating its antibacterial effects against the bad bacterias Bacillus subtilis, Pseudomonas aeruginosa, Staphylococcus aureus (which causes tooth decay) and E. coli. The study found that Lonicera japonica extract exhibited excellent antibacterial effects for the treatment of infectious and bacterial diseases.

FOR PROTECTION AND PREVENTION

The Lianhua qingwen capsule (LH)
This formula has been recommended for improving the clinical cure rate of COVID-19 [4e]. A clinical trial involving 142 confirmed cases of COVID-19 that took the Lianhua Qingwen Formula for 2 weeks exhibited a 91.5 % recovery rate. 83.8 % of the patients showed improved upper respiratory functioning and 78.9 % recovered completely [4f] [4g]. The Lianhua qingwen capsule consists of 11 herbs including Fructus Forsythiae, Lonicera japonica, Ephedra sinensis, Semen Armeniacae Amarum, Isatis tinctoria, Rhizoma Dryopteridis Crassi Rhizomatis, Herba Houttuyniae, Agastache rugosa, Rheum palmatum, Radix et Rhizoma Rhodiolae Crenulatae, and Glycyrrhiza, along with menthol and a traditional Chinese mineral medicine, Gypsum fibrosum (*Jia et al., 2015*). It is used in the treatment of influenza [5].

Isatis tinctoria in detail
The main effective components of Isatis tinctoria are its alkaloids which exhibit anti-virus activities. Studies on mice have found that the alkaloids in Isatis tinctoria exert protective effects (on mice) that were indirectly infected with the influenza A virus (*He et al., 2014*).

In a randomized controlled trial with LH capsule in COVID19 [6], patients they received standard treatment alone or a combination of LH (*4 capsules, thrice daily*) for 14 days. The study found that the rate of symptoms (fever, fatigue, coughing) was reduced. In summary LH capsule reduced the clinical symptoms of COVID-19 (*Li et al., 2020*). In summary, LH capsule may help protect one against coronavirus and serve as novel strategy for fighting COVID-19.

RECOMMENDED HERBS FOR THE EARLY STAGES OF COVID-19 INFECTION

The two most popular prescribed herbs used in TCM during the early stages of the COVID-19 infection are -

1- Ma xing shi gan decoction (MXSG)
The MXSG decoction consists of a total of four herbs that includes Glycyrrhiza, Ephedra sinensis, Gypsum fibrosum and Semen armeniacae amarum. This formula is used for treating cough, lung heat and asthma.

2 - Gancao ganjiang decoction (GCGJ)
The GCGJ decoction formula is made up of 2 simple herbs. These include Rhizoma zingiberis and Radix glycyrrhizae. This formula is used for treating yang deficiency of the stomach and spleen, weak and frequent urination, cold hands and feet, a short and weak pulse and dizziness. It is also used for chest and back pain, epigastric pain, intestinal

pain, acid vomiting, abdominal drainage, menstrual abdominal pain and asthma etc [7].

The Banxia Huoxiang Decoction, The Dayuan Decoction and The Sanxiao Decoction
These decoctions were found to effectively remove lung heat and toxic Qi and for treating COVID-19 patients with mild symptoms [7a 7b 7c].

The Most Popular Herbs Prescribed during the COVID-19 Outbreak
A group of researchers (*Zhang D. et al., 2020*). performed an in-depth meta-analysis study regarding the herbs most widely distributed during the COVID-19 outbreak. Xiong et al. stated that the herbs most used were Liquoric Root (Glycyrrhiza glabra L.), Baical Skullcap Root (Scutellaria baicalensis Georgi), Bitter Apricot Seed (Prunus armeniaca L.) Forsythia Fruit and Pinellia Rhizome (*Li et al., 2020*). Their study concluded that Chinese herbal medicines were effective at halting the progression of disease from mild to critical. This in turn decreased the hospitalization rate and reduced hospital stay (*Li et al., 2020*) [7d].

HERBAL FORMULAS FOR THE TREATMENT OF SEVERE COVID-19 CASES

Shen-fu-tang combined with the su-he-xiang pill was the most frequently suggested herbal combination to treat severe stages of COVID-19, including Pneumonia [7d]. Xiang-sha-liu-junzitang was most frequently prescribed during the recovery phase of COVID-19 (*Ang et al., 2020*) [7a]. Both of these formulas can be used if you do not have access to Ephedra.

The Shen-fu-tang + su-he-xiang pill consists of the following herbs - Glycyrrhiza glabra L. rhizomes and roots + Liquidambar orientalis, Mill. oleoresins, Schisandra chinensis (Turcz.) Baill. fruits, Zingiber officinale Roscoe rhizomes, Panax ginseng C.A.Mey. roots, Aconitum carmichaelii Debeaux roots, Acorus calamus L. rhizomes, Curcuma longa L. rhizomes and Cornus officinalis Siebold with Zucc. pulps.

Xiang-sha-liu-junzitang consists of the following herbs and is used for recovery - Glycyrrhiza glabra rhizomes, and roots, preserved Astragalus propinquus Schischkin roots in honey, Atractylodes macrocephala Koidz. rhizomes, Wolfiporia extensa (Peck) Ginns sclerotia and Codonopsis pilosula (Franch.) Nannf. roots.

FOR TREATMENT

The most commonly prescribed herbs used to Treat COVID-19.

Of 31 prescriptions used in the COVID-19 Chinese diagnosis and treatment program in China [8], 72 Traditional Chinese Medicine (TCM) herbs were prescribed (*Zhang and Li, 2020*). The top 5 prescribed herbs were as follows -

1 - Glycyrrhiza (*19 times*)

2 - Poria cocos (*18 times*)

3 - Tangerine peel (*18 times*)

4 - Ophiopogon japonicus (*17 times*)

5 - Astragalus membranaceus (*16 times*)

Tangerine peel in detail

Flavonoids are the main medicinal component in Tangerine peel. Studies have found that extracts of Tangerine peel greatly inhibited the scavenging hydroxyl free radicals (•OH) and oxidation of lard. In vivo experiments demonstrated that water extracts of tangerine peels greatly inhibited lipid peroxidation in the heart, brain and liver tissues in mice. It also significantly enhanced SOD activity (*Jing et al., 2003*).

Astragalus

Studies by Yu Ping Feng found that Astragalus membranaceus and Yu Ping Feng were used in 13 disease prevention programs in Beijing and Tianjin for "reinforcing one's vital qi". In TCM terms this means it boosts the body's immune system.

The 10 most commonly prescribed herbs by Chinese province

Astragalus membranaceus, Glycyrrhizae uralensis, Saposhnikoviae divaricata, Rhizoma Atractylodis Macrocephalae, Fructus forsythia, Agastache rugosa, Atractylodis Rhizoma, Radix platycodonis, Lonicerae Japonicae Flos and Cyrtomium fortune J. Sm [8a] [8b].

The most frequently prescribed Herbal Combinations

A study found that 24 herbal combinations were used more than 70 times for treating COVID. The two most commonly mentioned herbs are Ephedra sinica Stapf followed and Prunus armeniaca L.

Ephedra sinica Stapf and Prunus armeniaca L are used to retire the lung meridian. These herbs return strength to the lungs, discharge depressed lung heat and relieve asthma [8c].

The top 10 active substances found in the most popular COVID-19 Herbal Treatments
Yufeng Huang et, al. stated in their research paper that the active compounds present in several TCM prescriptions included: quercetin, baicalein, kaempferol, luteolin, isorhamnetin, naringenin, ergosterol, wogonin, lonicerin and tussilagone [8d].

TCM and Western Therapy Combination Treatments

The Maxing Shigan Formula in Combination with Western COVID-19 Treatments
When the Maxing Shigan Formula was combined with conventional western medicine treatment in 40 common cases of COVID-19 for 1-week, the patients experienced a removal of fever (96.8 %), fatigue (100 %) and cough (81.8 %) [8e].

The Toujie Quwen Formula combined with Arbidol
Toujie Quwen granules have been used in hospital treatments in combination with Arbidol. This combination exerted positive effects during early the treatment stages of COVID-19 patients with a total success rate of 89.2 % (n = 37) [8f].

The Lianhua Qingwen Formula with Arbidol Hydrochloride
A study by Suliman Khan and colleagues discovered that a combination therapy of The Lianhua Qingwen Formula with Arbidol Hydrochloride for up to a week in 122 patients that exhibited mild COVID-19 symptoms, exhibited a 98 % recovery rate [8g].

A combination of Qingfei Paidu and Interferon
22 patients treated with the Qingfei Paidu decoction and

Interferon α-1b exhibited a total recovery rate of almost 100 %[8h].

The Shufeng Jiedu Formula

This is one of the more simple formulas. The formula removes damp, detoxifies and assists in returning strength to the lungs. 100 patients with mild COVID-19 symptoms (fatigue, fever and dry cough) showed a reduction in their symptoms after combination therapy with the Shufeng Jiedu Formula and Arbidol[8i]. The main herbs in the Shufeng Jiedu Formula include - Verbena officinalis L, Glycyrrhiza glabra L, Reynoutria japonica Houtt, Forsythia suspensa (Thunb.) Vahl, Isatis indigotica Fort, Bupleurum abchasicum Manden and Patrinia heterophylla Bunge. The formula is recommended for early stages of COVID that include depressed lung activity and obstructions of cardinalate.

These results of these studies suggest that TCM and western therapies can work together to create effective treatments for helping defeat COVID-19.

FOR TREATMENT

The Qingfei Paidu decoction

The Qingfei Paidu decoction comes from the Treatise on Febrile Diseases. It is designed to act upon various stages and viscera of dampness, water, phlegm and fluid (*Fan et al., 2020*). Making it suitable for treating COVID-19 (*damp toxin and dampness, affecting cold and dryness*).

The Qingfei Paidu decoction has been used to treat 214 confirmed cases of COVID-19. Three days is a course of treatment. The total effective rate is more than 90%, in which, more than 60% of patients have improved symptoms, and 30% have stable symptoms without aggravation. The Qingfei Paidu decoction was proven effective in multi-provincial clinical trials. Since this time it was selected as an overall general prescription for treating patients infected with COVID-19; including those in various stages [9].

The Qingfei Paidu decoction is composed of the following 21 herbs -

Radix Glycyrrhizae (Glycyrrhiza uralensis Fisch.; 6 g; baked), Semen Armeniacae Amarum (Prunus armeniaca L.; 9 g), Herba Ephedrae (Ephedra sinica Stapf; 9 g), Raw Gypsum (15-30 g; first decocted), Polyporus Umbellatus (Polyporus umbellaru (Pers.) Fr.; 9 g), Rhizoma Atractylodis Macrocephalae (Atractylodes macrocephala Koidz.; 9 g), Herba Asari (Asarum sieboldii Miq.; 6 g), Rhizoma Dioscoreae (Dioscorea oppositifolia L.; 12 g), Pericarpium Citri Reticulatae (Citrus aurantium L.; 6 g), Ramulus Cinnamomi (Cinnamomum cassia (L.) J.Presl; 9 g), Rhizoma Alismatis (Alisma plantago-aquatica Linn.; 9 g), Poria (Poria cocos (Schw.) Wolf.; 15 g), Radix Bupleuri (Bupleurum chinensis DC.; 16 g), Radix Scutellariae (Scutellaria baicalensis Georgi; 6 g), Radix Asteris (Aster tataricus Linn. f.; 9 g), Flos Farfarae (Tussilago farfara Linn.; 9 g), Rhizoma Belamcandae (Iris domestica (L.) Goldblatt & Mabb.; 9 g), Rhizome Pinelliae Preparata (Pinellia ternata (Thunb.) Breit.; 9 g; processed with ginger), Rhizoma Zingiberis Recens (Zingiber officinale Roscoe; 9 g) and Herba Pogostemonis (Pogostemon cablin (Blanco) Benth.; 9 g). This prescription is mainly composed of Maxing Shigan decoction, Shegan Mahuang decoction, Fructus Aurantii Immaturus (Citrus sinensis Osbeck; 6 g), Xiaochaihu decoction and Wuling powder. The formula also incorporates the Daqinglong decoction, Juzhijiang decoction and the Fuling Xingren Gancao decoction.

FOR TREATMENT

These formulas have been used as a first line of defense treatment in Traditional Chinese Medicine hospitals of Wuhan, China.

The Qingfeipaidu decoction (QFPD)
The Qingfeipaidu decoction consists of a combination of 21 herbs that have been especially utilized for the treatment of exogenous diseases that cause cold pathogenic factors. The formula is found in the "Treatise on Febrile and Miscellaneous Diseases nowadays" (*Shang Han Za Bing Lun*). The formula has been designed for the early, lightly, and heavily stages of COVID-19 infected patients [10]. This formulas was also recommended for critical patients. The overall success rate of this formula was shown to be 92% (*Zhao et al., 2020*).

The herbs include Ephedra sinensis, Radix Glycyrrhizae, Rhizoma Alismatis, Polyporus umbellatus, Semen Armeniacae Amarum, Gypsum fibrosum, Pinelliae Rhizoma Praeparatum Cum Zingibere, Rhizoma Zingiberis Recens, Herba Asari, Yam, Immature bitter orange, Tangerine peel, Radix Asteris, Flos Farfarae, Ramulus Cinnamomi, Bupleurum chinense, Scutellaria baicalensis, Atractylodes macrocephala, Poria cocos, Rhizoma Belamcandae and Agastache rugosa (*Chen J, 2020a; Yang et al., 2020b*).

The herbal formula includes the maxingshigan decoction, the xiaochaihu decoction, wuling powder and the sheganmahuang decoction. Among the herbs listed Ziziphus jujuba, Ginseng and Schisandra chinensis seeds were removed and yam, tangerine peel, immature bitter orange and Agastache rugose were added.

Agastache rugosa in detail
Agastache rugosa has been scientifically proven to greatly inhibit replication of the H1N1 influenza virus in vitro (*Wu et al., 2013*). In mice studies, that were infected with lethal levels of FM1, the substance patchouli alcohol (methanol extract) was shown to significantly improve the survival rate of the mice. It also prolonged the mices' survival that were infected with influenza. During this trial it also significantly reduced the mices' inflammation of their lungs. Patchouli alcohol is extracted from Agastache rugosa (*Kiyohara et al., 2012*). The study found that the reduction of inflammation was due to the patchouli alcohol being able to regulate the inflammatory cytokines in the lung (*Li et al., 2012*). The study also found that the antiviral effect of the patchouli oil (in vitro) was anti-adenovirus. This may been what caused it to prevent the virus from adsorbing itself into the body's cells and causing illness (*Wei et al., 2013*).

FOR TREATMENT

A report documenting 73 patients infected with COVID-19 (*Yan et al., 2020*) stated that 24 herbs were used a total of 30 times [11]. The top 3 herbs prescribed in this report were as follows -

1 - Glycyrrhiza (4.28%)

2 - Scutellaria baicalensis (4.11%)

3 - Tangerine peel (3.37%)

Scutellaria baicalensis in detail
Baicalin and baicalin found in Scutellaria baicalensis has been shown to inhibit the growth of numerous Gram-positive and negative bacteria. Scutellaria baicalensis has

been shown to exhibit strong antiviral and antibacterial effects as well as significantly reduce pathogenic skin fungus bacteria (*Li, 2018*).

Scutellaria baicalensis exhibited excellent antiviral and antibacterial effects as well as significantly inhibited pathogenic skin fungus bacteria and reduced the growth of the Acinetobacter calcium acetate ndm-1 strain. It was also shown to effectively eliminate the drug-resistant plasmids. The best extraction method that yielded the best results was the alcohol extraction method, as it was found to be effective against the transmission of clinical infections of the hyperresistant Acinetobacter (*Liu et al., 2017*).

A research study looked at anti-SARS-CoV-2 activity of S. baicalensis and discovered that an ethanol extract of it (*with its major component being baicalein*) inhibited SARS-CoV-2 3CLpro activity in vitro at IC50's of 8.52mg/ml and 0.39 mM, respectively with the Baicalein showing its effectiveness at the very beginning stages of post-viral entry [11a].

FOR TREATMENT

A similar study involving 93 medicinal herbs prescribed for various TCM prescriptions for treating COVID-19 (*Shi et al., 2020*) showed that the top 10 prescribed herbs were -

1 - Astragalus membranaceus	6 - Tangerine peel
2 - Saposhniovia divaricata root	7 - Atractylodes lancea
3 - Glycyrrhiza	8 - Agastache rugosa
4 - Atractylodes macrocephala	9 - Platycodon grandiflorus
5 - Honeysuckle	10 - Fructus Forsythiae

Du et al. (*2017*) found that Honeysuckle inhibited the over expression of parasitoid interferon achieving anti-viral effects and avoiding inflammation and tissue damage [12].

Honeysuckle (Flos Lonicerae Japonicae) in detail
Honeysuckle (Flos Lonicerae Japonicae). This plant has been shown to exhibit a broad range of antiviral effects on the influenza virus, the avian influenza virus H9 subtype (H9-AIV), enterovirus EV71, the respiratory syncytial virus (RSV), the herpes virus and others.. (*Liu et al., 2020b*).

An alcohol extract of Honeysuckle has been shown to significantly reduce ear swelling that has been caused by xylene as well as foot swelling caused by carrageenin in studies conducted on mice (with the results being dose-dependent manner) (*Zhang and Chen, 2019*).

FOR TREATMENT

In an in-depth analysis of prescribed treatment involving a total of 875 patients a combined total of 233 Traditional Chinese Medicinal herbs were used. The most frequently used herb was Scutellaria baicalensis (*Chen et al., 2020)*. The top 12 herbs are as follows -

1 - Scutellaria baicalensis	8 - Yam
2 - Fructus Forsythiae	9 - Radix Glycyrrhizae
3 - Rhizoma Belamcandae	10 - Platycodon grandiflorus
4 - Agastache rugosa	11- Poria cocos
5 - Glycyrrhiza	12- Herba Menthae
6 - Szechuan fritillary bulb	Haplocalycis
7 - Semen Armeniacae Amarum	

Scutellaria for pneumonia

Research studies have found that lung tissue is repaired by the herb Scutellaria baicalensis Georgi. Its mechanism of action works by reducing levels of TNF-α, IL-1 and IL-6. It has been recommended for the treatment of Pneumonia [12a].

FOR TREATMENT

In a statistical analysis of medicinal herbs prescribed for 149 prescriptions, 14 were prescribed over 30 times (*Cheng et al.,2020*). These were as follows –

1 – Glycyrrhiza	9 – Ginseng
2 – Semen Armeniacae	10 – Poria cocos
3 – Amarum	11 – Astragalus membranaceus
4 – Ephedra sinensis	12 – Lonicera japonica
5 – Tangerine peel	13 – Pinelliae Rhizoma Praeparatum Cum Zingibere
6 – Gypsum fibrosum	
7 – Atractylodes lancea	14 – Atractylodes macrocephala
8 – Agastache rugosa	15 – Scutellaria baicalensis

FOR TREATMENT

Out of 76 medicinal herbs used in 30 TCM formulas for treating patients diagnosed with COVID-19 in China, the following were used with the most frequently prescribed herbs shown first [13] –

1 – Glycyrrhiza (*17 times*)	8 – Ramulus Cinnamomi (*7 times*)
2 – Scutellaria baicalensis (*11 times*)	9 – Semen Armeniacae Amarum (*5 times*)
3 – Rhizoma Zingiberis Recens (*11 times*)	10 – Ginseng (*5 times*)
4 – Paeonia lactiflora root (*9	11 – Bupleurum chinense (*5

times)	times)
5 - Ziziphus jujube (*9 times*)	12 - Gypsum fibrosum (Sheng Shi Gao) (*5 times*)
6 - Pinelliae Rhizoma Praeparatum Cum Zingibere (*8 times*)	13 - Platycodon grandiflorus (*5 times*)
7 - Ephedra sinensis (*7 times*)	14 - Magnolia officinalis (*5 times*)

Magnolia officinalis (Rehder) in detail
Magnolol, found in Magnolia bark, has been identified as a potential enhancer of ACE2 expression (*ANSES, 2020*). This makes it a possible candiate for controlling or preventing COVID-19.

TCM Preparations for Enhancing Immune System Functioning in Patients with COVID-19

Maxingshigan decoction (MXSG)
MXSG decoction improved the immune function of the body regulated the expression and secretion of cytokines, thereby reducing lung inflammation and improving the general condition of influenza virus pneumonia in animal studies (*Li et al., 2018*).

The MXSG decoction down-regulated the secretion and protein expression levels of IFNα and IFN-β macrophages infected with influenza virus and played an antiviral role (*Zhang et al., 2019*). The MXSG decoction also protected against acute lung injury caused by influenza virus infection The MXSG decoction also improved the immune system of the body, up-regulated the protein expression and secretion levels of IL-2 and IL-4, and down-regulated the protein expression and secretion levels of TNF to treat viral pneumonia (*Li et al., 2018*). In addition, MXSG decoction significantly reduced the pulmonary inflammation in vivo as evidenced by pathological examination. MXSG decoction attenuated the LPS-induced inflammation in lung tissues. It is conceivable that MXSG decoction acts on COVID-19 by targeting IL-6, TNF-α, MAPK-8, MAPK-3, CASP-3, TP53, IL-10, CXCL-8, MAPK-1, CCL-2, IL-1β, IL-4 and PTGS-2. Among them, IL-6 is currently a clinical early-warning indicator for severe COVID-19 diagnosis and one of the major therapeutic targets.

FOR RECOVERY AND TREATMENT

During the recovery stage, lymphocyte count is increased [13a] and a number of natural killer T cells (NKT) go into decline. This is because the body's T cells are giving themselves up to clear the virus as the initial infection slowly dies [13b].

During recovery the qi-deficiency in the spleen and lung show improvement. This is motivated by a herbal formula consisting of Astragali Radix preparata, Codonopsis pilosula, Atractylodes macrocephala Koidz, Pinellinae Rhizoma Praeparata, Citrus reticulata Blanco, Poria cocos, Pogostemon cablin, Glycyrrhiza uralensis Fisch and Amomum villosum Lour [13c].

FOR RECOVERY AND TREATMENT

The Sheganmahuang decoction (SMD)
This formula is designed to Relieve Asthma and reduce Airway Restriction. The Sheganmahuang Decoction is made up of 9 herbs. These herbs include Schisandra chinensis seeds, Asarum sieboldii, Radix Asteris, Flos Farfarae, Rhizoma Belamcandae, Ephedra sinensis Rhizoma Zingiberis Recens, Ziziphus jujube and Pinelliae Rhizoma Praeparatum Cum Zingibere.

These herbs have been scientifically proven to relieve

asthma and reduce airway restriction. It not only helpful to dispel heat and reduce poison, but its active ingredients have significant anti-inflammatory and antiviral effects (*Eng et al., 2019*). SMD is also used to treat bronchial asthma by regulating immune inflammatory pathways (*Lin et al., 2020*).

Jinhuaqinggan granules (JHQG)
Studies on Jinhua Qinggan Granules showed that they significantly reduced cytokines in serum, enhanced the immune system and exhibited significant therapeutic effects [13d] [13e]. These granules may significantly alleviate clinical symptoms associated with COVID-19 such as fever, cough, expectoration, fatigue as well as relieve the psychological anxiety that manifests in patients diagnosed with COVID-19. The Jinhua Qinggan Granules were originally developed during the 2009 H1N1 influenza pandemic. The formula consists of 12 herbs. These are Mahuang (Ephedrae Herba), Huangqin (Scutellariae Radix), Lianqiao (Forsythiae Fructus), Jinyinhua (Lonicerae Japonicae Flos), Shigao (Gypsum Fibrosum), Qinghao (Artemisiae Annuae Herba), Bohe (Menthae Haplocalycis Herba), Kuxingren (Armeniacae Semen Amarum), Zhebeimu (Fritillariae Thunbergii Bulbus), Gancao (Glycyrrhizae Radix et Rhizoma), Zhimu (Anemarrhenae Rhizoma) and Niubangzi (Arctii Fructus).

The Jinhua Qinggan Granules are used for treating pneumonia, fever, sore throat, stuffy nose, thirst, coughing or coughing with phlegm [14]. JHQG granules consists of Maxingshigan decoction and Yinqiao San, which is composed of Honeysuckle, Ephedra sinensis, Gypsum fibrosum, Semen Armeniacae Amarum, Scutellaria baicalensis, Fructus Forsythiae, Bulbus Fritillariae Thunbergii, Rhizoma Anemarrhenae, Fructus Arctii, Herba Artemisiae Annuae, Herba Menthae Haplocalycis, Glycyrrhiza. (*Liu et al., 2020*). An extract of Fructus

Forsythiae reduced the mortality of mice infected with influenza virus, prolonged the survival time and significantly improved the symptoms of pneumonia in mice. The activity of influenza A virus was significantly reduced in vitro (*Pu et al., 2010*).

FOR RECOVERY

Shengmai san and Ginseng were the most frequently prescribed herbs. Ginseng is used to assist patients in a speedy recovery. Shengmai san improves blood circulation as well as heart function. Hence, healthy blood circulation enhances one's recovery from lung damage by improving the microcirculation of each of the lungs' cells [15].

Radix Rehmanniae

Radix Rehmanniae is commonly used in numerous TCM formulas for treating various viral infections. Catalpol is an iridoid glycoside that is extracted from the pure roots of Rehmannia. Catalpol has been reported to protect against LPS-induced acute lung injury via the Toll-like receptor-4 (TLR-4)-mediated NF-kB signaling pathway (*Ma et al., 2014*). Catalpol has also demonstrated excellent behavior for supporting the clinical efficacy of Radix Rehmanniae for treating COVID-19 patients that have been admitted to the ICU [15a].

Recommended Herbs for Prevention and Treatment by the Country of India (AYUSH)

Ayurveda treatments aim to create healing in the body by targeting healing activators in the body's immune system (mediated by psychoneuroimmune mechanisms and the meaning response (*Golechha, 2020; Rajkumar, 2020*). Indian Medicinal plants used to boost the immune system include - Withania somnifera (L.) Dunal, Allium sativum L., Cinnamomum verum J.Presl, Cuminum cyminum L., Curcuma longa L., Ocimum tenuiflorum L., and Zingiber officinale Roscoe. All these herb exhibit immunomodulatory properties in the form of single herbal mixture (*Sheoran et al., 2017; Subhrajyoti & Shalini, 2020; Tabarsa et al., 2020*).

Clinical research settings and the regulations COVID-19 treatment using Ayurveda, Siddha, Unani and Homeopathy systems or people living in India are available for review by the Indian Ministry of Ayush (*INDIA, 2020*).

The Ministry of AYUSH (*Ayurvedic, Yoga and Naturopathy, Unani, Siddha and Homeopathy*) recommended to its citizens to consume the drink called Kadha in order to boost immunity (*AYUSH Advisory, 2020*). Kadha is prepared from certain herbs and spices [16].

Medicinal plants recommended for the prevention and prophylactic of COVID-19 include the warm extracts of the following -

For chronic fever - Tinospora cordifolia

For fever and cold - Andrograhis paniculata

For enhancing immune-modulatory and influenza resistance - Cydonia oblonga, Zizyphus jujube and Cordia myxa and Arsenicum album 30 (*found effective against SARS-CoV-2, immune-modulator*).

Agastya Haritaki (*and sesame oil drops*) has been suggested for the management of patients diagnosed with COVID-19 to help prevent upper respiratory infections (*Vellingiri et al., 2020*).

A Spice Combo
A mixture of lavanga (Syzygium aromaticum), sunthi (Zingiber officinale Roscoe.) and maricha (Piper nigrum) was recommended for people wanting to avoid contracting COVID-19 as well as person's infected with COVID-19. as it has shown the ability to provide support in the cell and humoral mediated responses, as well as enhances breathing passages [17].

Plants like thyme, cinnamon, star anise, oregano, garlic, mint, tulsi, fennel, ginger, lemon and broccoli may also hold potential substances to fight COVID-19 (*Yasmin et al., 2020*).

Curcuma xanthorrhiza (curumin) for reducing cytokine storms

Curcuma xanthorrhiza (curumin)
Xanthorrhizol is found in Java turmeric or Curcuma xanthorrhiza. Java turmeric comes from Indonesia and grows wild in the Philippines, Sri Lanka, Thailand and Malaysia where it is used to enhance the taste of food.

A research study showed that Xanthorrhizol decreased inflammatory genes in the body's liver, adipose tissue and muscles in patients diagnosed with diabetes mellitus. Hence, Xanthorrhizol may restore balance to the immune system by reducing cytokine storms [18].

Another study suggested Xanthorrhizol increased serum transforming growth factor (TGFβ) as well as decreased serum levels of IL-6 in patients with SLE with hypovitamin D [19].

Another study found that Xanthorrhizol promoted the production of anti-inflammatory cytokines and inhibits proinflammatory cytokines [20].

Does Vitamin D3 help protect against COVID-19?
While Vitamin D shows good protection, Vitamin D3 does not. Out of 240 hospitalized COVID-19 patients, the patients who took a single high dose of vitamin D3 did not experience a significant reduction in hospital stay [21a].

Xanthorrhizol Summary
Because Xanthorrhizol acts as an immunosuppressant, it may find use as a treatment for COVID-19 patients because it inhibits proinflammatory cytokines. Patients diagnosed with COVID-19 are susceptible to such a condition. Hence, Xanthorrhizol may lower the proinflammatory response.

Curcuma xanthorrhiza has been shown to block cytokine release (interleukin-1, interleukin-6), thus reducing the body's susceptibility to a cytokine storm, keeping the immune system healthy [22]. It is commonly consumed with milk (*Omara et al., 2010*).

Further Reading
Potential effects of curcumin in the treatment of COVID-19 infection. Phytother. Res. 1-10. doi: 10.1002/ptr.6738. Zahedipour, F et al. (2020).

Nano curcumin significantly reduces fever and cough
In herbology, the best way to get the most out of a herb is to know how to properly prepare and deliver it. Different herbs have different methods of preparation and delivery.

Certain herbs work extremely well when properly prepared. For example, if you put Goji berries in a pot and bring them to a moderate boil, their antioxidant levels will increase substantially. I list this fact in further detail in my latest anti-aging book. Curcumin when delivered in nano sized form was tested in patients that were hospitalized with mild to moderate COVID-19. After 2 weeks, the majority of symptoms such as fever and cough were significantly reduced in the curcumin group compared to the control group. Also hospital stays were shorter. The study also stated no patient in the group taking the nano-sized curcumin experienced a deterioration in their infection during the follow-up; however it occurred in 40% of the control group. The researchers concluded that oral curcumin in nano-form significantly improves recovery time for hospitalized COVID-19 patients.

Further Reading
Curcumin, a traditional spice component, can it hold the promise against COVID-19? Vivek Kumar Soni et al. November 2020.

Ayurveda Practitioners advise for early-stage patients diagnosed with COVID-19 the following herbs - Glycyrrhiza glabra L. (Fabaceae), Adhatoda vasica Ness (Acanthaceae), (Acanthaceae), Zingiber officinale Roscoe (Zingiberaceae), Curcuma longa L.(Zingiberaceae), Swertia chirata Buch.-Ham. ex Wall. (Gentianaceae), Terminalia bellirica (Gaertn.) Roxb. (Combretaceae), Tinospora cordifolia (Willd.) Myers (Menispermaceae), Ocimum sanctum L. (Lamiaceae), Moringa oleifera Lam (Moringaceae), Triphala [a mixture of the dried fruits of Emblica officinalis Gaertn. (Phyllanthaceae), Andrographis paniculata (Burm.f.) (Acanthaceae), Terminalia chebula Retz.(Combretaceae)] and Trikatu [a complementary formula to Triphala, including Piper nigrum L. (Piperaceae), Piper longum L. (Piperaceae) as well as Z. officinale Roscoe] (*Rastogi et al., 2020*).

Indonesian Herbs used to Fight COVID-19
The Indonesian Government has suggested the use of certain medicinal plants that behave as immunostimulatory agents to help defeat COVID-19. These plants include - Curcuma zanthorrhiza, Psidium guajava L, Phyllantus niruri L, Zingiber officinale Roscoe var Rubrum and Andrographis paniculata (Burm.f.) Nees (*Indonesian NADFC, 2020d*)

Further Reading
The Potential Roles of Jamu for COVID-19: A Learn from the Traditional Chinese Medicine. Dwi Hartanti et al. June 2020.

Turkish Folk Medicinal Herbs used for treating COVID-10
Turkey has a rich history of herbal use for the treatment and the prevention of influenza. A research study examined 224 herbs belonging to 45 species of plants that were associated with 81 studies in seven regions of the country of Turkey [23]. Out of these just 35 (15.6%) were subjected to research studies (in vitro and in vivo) for their anti-influenza activity. Out of 56 active substances identified in Turkish herbs used in folk medicine, the substances Quercetin and Chlorogenic acid were identified as the most common (7.1%) active ingredients. As far as the most common plants used, Rosa canina (58.7%) and Mentha x piperita (22.2%) were the most common plants used in Turkey to fight influenza and associated diseases. Other species included Sambucus nigra (11.6%), Eucalyptus spp., Melissa officinalis, Origanum vulgare (7.0%) and Olea

europaea (9.3%), were the most investigated taxa. Regarding malaria, the Turkish plant Centaurea drabifolia subsp. Phlocosa was been found to be effective for treating malaria. In conclusion, 39 Turkish plants are confirmed for their anti-influenza activity, which are a rich source of pharmacological substances. Also there are potential discoveries waiting to be unveiled with the remaining 189 species of plants (84.4%); allowing pharmacological researchers a ground floor opportunity to exploit these plants for their potential for anti-influenza activity.

A Herbal COVID-19 Resistance Formula for the Elderly. The Eight-Section Brocade

Before I conclude this chapter, I would like to share a study that has shown positive benefit in elderly people who have COVID-19. Lulu Zha et, al. [24] stated a reduction in cough and expectoration was observed after 60 elderly patients with mild symptoms of COVID-19 took the Eight-Section Brocade formula (a median age of 54 years old).

Numerical References. Chapter 5

(1) Research Advance on Qingfei Paidu Decoction in Prescription Principle, Mechanism Analysis and Clinical Application. www.frontiersin.org. Wei Ren et al. Jan 2021.

(1a) X.Y. Fan, Z. Hao, Preventive treatment of disease in dietetic therapy based on Qianjin Fang, Journal of Changchun University of Chinese Medicine. 36 (6) (2020) 1107-1110.

(1b) D. Wang, K.J. Yin, K.H. Ren, Discussion on SUN Si-miao's contribution to acupuncture and moxibustion medicine, Chinese Journal of Traditional Chinese Medicine. 35 (7) (2020) 3734-3736.

(1c) Traditional Chinese Medicine treatment of COVID-19. Jia Xu* and Yunfei Zhang. May 2020.

(1d) Traditional Chinese Medicine treatment of COVID-19. Jia Xu* and Yunfei Zhang. May 2020.

(2) Cinatl, J.; Morgenstern, B.; Bauer, G.; Chandra, P.; Rabenau, H.; Doerr, H.W. Glycyrrhizin, an active component of liquorice roots, and replication of SARS-associated coronavirus. Lancet 2003, 361, 2045-2046.

(3) Huan, C.-C.; Wang, H.-X.; Sheng, X.-X.; Wang, R.; Wang, X.; Mao, X. Glycyrrhizin inhibits porcine epidemic diarrhea virus infection and attenuates the proinflammatory responses by inhibition of high mobility group box-1 protein. Arch. Virol. 2017, 162, 1467-1476.

(4) Michaelis, M.; Geiler, J.; Naczk, P.; Sithisarn, P.; Leutz, A.; Doerr, H.W.; Cinatl, J. Glycyrrhizin Exerts Antioxidative Effects in H5N1 Influenza A Virus-Infected Cells and Inhibits Virus Replication and Pro-Inflammatory Gene Expression. PLoSONE 2011, 6, e19705.

(4a) (Ho, T.-Y.; Wu, S.-L.; Chen, J.-C.; Li, C.-C.; Hsiang, C.-Y. Emodin blocks the SARS coronavirus spike protein and angiotens in converting enzyme 2 interaction. Antivir. Res. 2007, 74, 92–101)

(4b) R.Q. Wang, S.J. Yang, C.G. Xie, Q.L. Shen, M.Q. Li, X. Lei, J.K. Li, M. Huang, Clinical observation of qingfeipaidu decoction in the treatment of COVID-19, Pharmacology and Clinics of Chinese Materia Medica. 36 (1) (2020) 13–18.

(4c) Potential Targets for Treatment of Coronavirus Disease 2019 (COVID-19): A Review of Qing-Fei-Pai-Du-Tang and Its Major Herbs. Linda Li et al.

(4d) Analysis on herbal medicines utilized for treatment of COVID-19. Lu Luoa. et al .July 2020.

(4e) Mechanism and material basis of Lianhua Qingwen capsule for improving clinical cure rate of COVID-19: a study based on network pharmacology and molecular docking technology. Haiyan Yan et al. Jan 2021.Journal of Southern Medical University 2021 January 30, 41 (1): 20-30.

(4f) Traditional Chinese herbal medicine at the forefront battle against COVID19: Clinical experience and scientific basis (David Y.W. Lee et al. Sept 2020).

(4g) K. Hu, W.J. Guan, Y. Bi, W. Zhang, L. Li, B. Zhang, Q. Liu, Y. Song, X. Li, Z. Duan, Q. Zheng, Z. Yang, J. Liang, M. Han, L. Ruan, C. Wu, Y. Zhang, Z.H. Jia, N. S. Zhong, Efficacy and safety of Lianhuaqingwen capsules, a repurposed Chinese herb, in patients with coronavirus disease 2019: a multicenter, prospective, randomized controlled trial, Phytomedicine (2020), 153242..

(5) Traditional Chinese herbal medicine at the forefront battle against COVID19: Clinical experience and scientific basis (David Y.W. Lee et al. Sept 2020.

(6) Traditional Chinese herbal medicine at the forefront battle against COVID19: Clinical experience and scientific basis (David Y.W. Lee et al. Sept 2020).

(7) Traditional Chinese herbal medicine at the forefront battle against COVID19: Clinical experience and scientific basis (David Y.W. Lee et al. Sept 2020.

(7a) Z. Zhao, Y. Li, L. Zhou, X. Zhou, B. Xie, W. Zhang, J. Sun, Prevention and treatment of COVID-19 using Traditional Chinese medicine: a review, Phytomedicine (2020), 153308.

(7b) H.A. He, X. Wang, Z. Song, B.Q. ZHang, Study on the molecular mechanism of Sanxiao decoction in the treatment of novel coronavirus pneumonia, Journal of Chinese Medicinal Materials. 43 (7) (2020) 1772-1776.

(7c) X. Ruan, P. Du, K. Zhao, J. Huang, H. Xia, D. Dai, S. Huang, X. Cui, L. Liu, J. Zhang, Mechanism of Dayuanyin in the treatment of coronavirus disease 2019 based on network pharmacology and molecular docking, Chin. Med. 15 (2020).

(7d) The Potential Roles of Jamu for COVID-19: A Learn from the Traditional Chinese Medicine. Dwi Hartanti et al. June 2020.

(7e) Current Prevention of COVID-19: Natural Products and Herbal Medicine. Junqing Huang et al. Oct 2020.

(8) Traditional Chinese herbal medicine at the forefront battle against COVID19: Clinical experience and scientific basis (David Y.W. Lee et al. Sept 2020.

(8a) Can Chinese Medicine Be Used for Prevention of Corona Virus Disease 2019 (COVID-19)? A Review of Historical Classics, Research Evidence and Current Prevention Programs. Luo H et al. Chin J Integr Med. 2020.

(8b) Xu X, Zhang Y, Li X, Li XX. Analysis on prevention plan of corona virus disease-19 (COVID-19) by traditional Chinese medicine in various regions. Chin Herb Med. 2020: 1-7.

(8c) Research progress of traditional Chinese medicine against COVID-19. Wei Ren et al. February 2021.

(8d) Y.F. Huang, C. Bai, F. He, Y. Xie, H. Zhou, Review on the potential action mechanisms of Chinese medicines in treating Coronavirus Disease 2019, COVID19), Pharmacological Research. 158 (2020), 104939.

(8e) Research progress of traditional Chinese medicine against COVID-19. Wei Ren et al. February 2021.

(8f) X.X. Fu, L.P. Lin, X.H. Tan, Clinical study on 37 case of COVID-19 treated with integrated traditional Chinese and western medicine, Traditional Chinese Drug Research & Clinical Pharmacology 31 (5) (2020) 600–604.

(8g) S.L. Khan, A. Ali, H.W. Shi, R. Siddique, Shabana, G. Nabi, J.J. Hu, T.J. Wang, M. Dong, W.J. Zaman, G. Han, COVID-19: Clinical aspects and therapeutics responses, J. Saudi Pharm. Soc. 28 (8) (2020) 1004–1008.

(8h) J. Liu, D.M. Yang, Z. Li, C. Yang, Clinical characteristics of 22 cases of COVID-19 and analysis of the combination of Chinese and Western Medicine, Journal of MuDanJiang Medical University 41 (4) (2020) 42–44.

(8i) Research progress of traditional Chinese medicine against COVID-19. Wei Ren et al. February 2021.

(9) Research Advance on Qingfei Paidu Decoction in Prescription Principle, Mechanism Analysis and Clinical Application. www.frontiersin.org. Wei Ren et al. Jan 2021.

(10) Research Advance on Qingfei Paidu Decoction in Prescription Principle, Mechanism Analysis and Clinical Application. www.frontiersin.org. Wei Ren et al. Jan 2021.

(11) Research Advance on Qingfei Paidu Decoction in Prescription Principle, Mechanism Analysis and Clinical Application. www.frontiersin.org. Wei Ren et al. Jan 2021.

(11a) Herbal immune-boosters: Substantial warriors of pandemic Covid-19 battle. Kanika Khannaa et al. Sept 2020.

(12) Traditional Chinese herbal medicine at the forefront battle against COVID19: Clinical experience and scientific basis. David Y.W. Lee et al. Sept 2020.

(12a) H.R. Xu, Y.L. Li, C.X. Wang, G.X. Liu, C. Liu, Effect of Scutellariae Radix on expression of inflammatory cytokine protein and gene in lung of mice with viral pneumonia caused by influenza virus FM1 infection, Chinese Journal of Traditional Chinese Medicine. 44 (23) (2019) 5166–5173.

(13) Research Advance on Qingfei Paidu Decoction in Prescription Principle, Mechanism Analysis and Clinical Application. www.frontiersin.org. Wei Ren et al. Jan 2021.

(13a) T. Ahmad, R. Chaudhuri, M.C. Joshi, A. Almatroudi, A.H. Rahmani, S.M. Ali, COVID-19: The Emerging Immunopathological Determinants for Recovery or Death, Front. Microbiol. 11 (11) (2020), 588409.

(13b) T. Ahmad, R. Chaudhuri, M.C. Joshi, A. Almatroudi, A.H. Rahmani, S.M. Ali, COVID-19: The Emerging Immunopathological Determinants for Recovery or Death, Front. Microbiol. 11 (11) (2020), 588409.

(13c) Research progress of traditional Chinese medicine against COVID-19. Wei Ren et al. February 2021.

(13d) Duan C. Clinical observation of novel coronavirus infected pneumonia treated by Jinhua Qinggan Granule. J. Tradit. Chinese Med. 2020:1–5.

(13e) Reflections on treatment of COVID-19 with traditional Chinese medicine. Hua Luo et al. Sept 2020.

(14) Traditional Chinese herbal medicine at the forefront battle against COVID19: Clinical experience and scientific basis. David Y.W. Lee et al. Sept 2020.

(15) Traditional Chinese herbal medicine at the forefront battle against COVID19: Clinical experience and scientific basis. David Y.W. Lee et al. Sept 2020.

(15a) Traditional Chinese herbal medicine at the forefront battle against COVID19: Clinical experience and scientific basis. David Y.W. Lee et al. Sept 2020.

(16) Herbal immune-boosters: Substantial warriors of pandemic Covid-19 battle. Kanika Khannaa et al. Sept 2020.

(17) Carrasco et al., 2009; Kim and Lee, 2009; Bui et al., 2019), (Herbal immune-boosters: Substantial warriors of pandemic Covid-19 battle. Kanika Khannaa et al. Sept 2020.

(18) Vander Hoek, L.; Pyrc, K.; Berkhout, B. Human corona virus NL63, a new respiratory virus. FEMS Microbiol. Rev. 2006,30,760–773.

(19) C. Singgih Wahono, C. Diah Setyorini, H. Kalim, N. Nurdiana, and K. Handono, "Effect of Curcuma xanthorrhiza supplementation on systemic lupus erythematosus patients with hypovitamin D which were given vitamin D3 towards disease activity (SLEDAI),IL-6,andTGF-β1serum," International Journal of Rheumatology, vol. 2017, Article ID 7687053, 8 pages, 2017.

(20) M.-B. Kim, C. Kim, Y. Song, and J.-K. Hwang, "Antihyperglycemic and anti-inflammatory effects of standardized Curcuma xanthorrhiza Roxb extract and its active compound xanthorrhizol in high fat diet induced obese mice." EvidenceBased Complementary and Alternative Medicine, vol. 2014, Article ID 205915, 10 pages, 2014.

(21) Seven recommendations to rescue the patients and reduce the mortality from COVID-19 infection: An immunological point of view. Andreas Kronbichler et al. May 2020.

(21a) Effect of a Single High Dose of Vitamin D3 on Hospital Length of Stay in Patients With Moderate to Severe COVID-19: A Randomized Clinical Trial. Igor H Murai et al. March 2021.

(22) Oral nano-curcumin formulation efficacy in management of mild to moderate hospitalized coronavirus disease-19 patients: An open label nonrandomized clinical trial. Jan 2021.

(23) Potential anti-influenza effective plants used in Turkish folk medicine: A review. Seyid Ahmet Sargin et al. Journal of Ethnopharmacology 2021 January 30, 265: 113319.

(24) L. Zha, X. Xu, D. Wang, G. Qiao, W. Zhuang, S. Huang, Modified rehabilitation exercises for mild cases of COVID-19, Ann. Palliat. Med. 9 (5) (2020) 3100–3106.

Chapter 6. Interviews with Professional Herbalists and their recommend Herbs for Treating and Preventing COVID-19

A research study titled: *COVID-19, prevention and treatment with herbal medicine in the herbal markets of Salé Prefecture, North-Western Morocco* that was published in 2021 by Noureddine C and colleagues in The European Journal of Integrative Medicine lists the results of in-person interviews with professional Herbalists in Salé Prefecture in the country of Morocco from March 1st, 2020 to May 31st, 2020.

All the herbalists stated they acquired their traditional knowledge of herbs and their preparation from their parents, friends, and elderly relatives, with 41.18% of the herbalists having experience as herbalists for more than 20 years.

Plant Species
The study consisted of face to face interviews with 30 known herbalists. The data included in the study looked at 20 plant species from 20 genera and 14 families which were used most frequently by the herbalists for the treatment and prevention of COVID 19.

Most Common Plants used to Treat COVID-19
The plant most mentioned was Eucalyptus globulus Labill.; followed by Azadirachta indica A. Juss and Ziziphus lotus (L.) Lam. In a research study titled: *Small molecules targeting severe acute respiratory syndrome human*

coronavirus that was conducted by Wu CY and colleagues and published in July 2004, the authors stated that extracts of eucalyptus as well as Lonicera japonica have been shown to inhibit SARS-CoV replication at non-toxic concentrations.

Plant Parts Used

The most commonly parts of the plant used were the leaves (28.43%) the seeds (17.5%), the whole plant (13%), the bulbs (11.27%), rhizomes (8.4%), other parts (7.6%), flowers (7%) and the fruits (6.8%). The majority of the remedies were prepared via infusions.

Solvents mixed with Herbs

The major solvent used in preparing the herbs was water; however tea, honey, milk, butter, cereal oils and vinegar, were equally extensively used ingredients.

Principal Preparations

The principal method of preparation reported was infusion (34.63%). The next most common method was decoction (25.1%) followed by powder (15.2%), and maceration (13.8%).

Infusions were the most common mentioned method (34.63%) for extracting the healing ingredients from the herb(s). Infusions make it possible to accumulate multiple effective healing components and eliminates some of the poisonous ingredients. Another popular method for extracting the healing substances from the herbs was via decoction.

Herbalist Age Grouping

Most herbalists interviewed were over 50 years of age. 17 were between the ages of 30 and 50. One was younger than thirty years old. More than half (53.3%) had a secondary education, 26.7% had a primary education, 16.7% were illiterate and 3.3% had graduate education.

Herbalists by Geographic Regions
Of the 30 herbalists interviewed, 33.33% were from Bab Lamrissa, 23.34% from Tabriquet, 20% from Laayayda, 13.33% from Bettana and 10% from Bouknadel.

Gender
Male participants accounted for 24 herbalists and female herbalists consisted of 6 herbalists.

Type of Plants
During the interviews, plants from the Lamiaceae family were most commonly mentioned (3 species,15%) for treating patients infected with COVID-19. The following are the herbs most used from most used to least used.

Eucalyptus globulus Labill. (MUV =0.967)

Azadirachta indica A. Juss. (MUV =0.933)

Ziziphus lotus (L.) Lam. (MUV =0.9)

These herbs and plants used in Morocco were found to be very similar to the plants and herbs used in Pakistan and other countries to treat patients infected with the COVID-19 virus.

Eucalyptus Oil
Eucalyptol, which comes from Eucalyptus globulus Labill. is identified as being an effective antiviral compound against coronavirus, with special emphasis on destroying the COVID-19 virus. This is due to the fact that the major

constituent of eucalyptus oil consists of hydroxyl (-OH) groups and ether (-O), ketones (=O). These play major roles in helping neutralize the SARS-CoV-2 virus [1].

Further Reading
Antiviral activity of tea tree and eucalyptus oil aerosol and vapour. Usachev E.V., Pyankov O.V., Usacheva O.V., Agranovski I.E. J. Aerosol Sci. 2013;59:22-30. doi: 10.1016/j.jaerosci.2013.01.004.

How does an Essential Oil Destroy Viruses?
Essential oils work their magic by inserting themselves into the lipid double layer (nonspecifically) of viral envelopes. This in turn alters the fluidity of the virus membrane [2] [3].

Essential Oils for Inhibiting COVID-19
Scientific analysis of the essential oils of lemon and geranium showed that these essential oils significantly downregulated ACE2, all without displaying cytotoxicity [3a]. The major components of lemon and geranium essential oil are; geraniol, limonene, linalool, citronellol and neryl acetate. Hence because of their ability to downregulate ACE2 expression in epithelial cells, they play a major role in blocking virus entry into host cells; thus preventing viral infection.

Herbs used in Steam Inhalation Therapy for combating COVID-19
Three common Indian herbs used steam inhalation therapy were researched for their effectiveness against COVID-19 [3b]. The researchers looked at the two main bioactives present in each popular plant.

Eucalyptus globulus - contained apigenin-o-7-glucuronide and ellagic acid

Vitex negundo - contained eudesmol and viridiflorene

Justicia adhatoda - contained vasicolinone and anisotine

These molecules were identified as the main substances responsible for helping treat sinus and related problems. Future research may reveal these help fight COVID-19.

The anti-viral activity exhibited by Terpenoids
An extensive search using Science Direct, PubMed, ISI, Google Scholar and Scopus using the words COVID-19, SARS and MERS and the words natural product, herb, plant, and extract. found that Zingiber officinale, Nigella sativa, Echinacea spp. Hypericum perforatum, Glycyrrhiza glabra, Scutellaria baicalensis, Allium sativum, Camellia sinensis improve the immune system [3c]. These herbs and plants are abundant in specific Terpenoids which show promising effects in viral replication inhibition. Also certain alkaloid structures such as lycorine, homoharringtonine and emetine exhibit powerful anti-coronavirus effects. Also specific herbs inhibit various coronavirus targets such as viral enzymes replication. These include 3CLpro (Iguesterin), helicase (Silvestrol), PLpro (Cryptotanshinone), RdRp (Sotetsuflavone) and S protein (emodin, baicalin). Hence these substances found in herbs and plants may act as powerful natural preventives as well as exhibit therapeutic effects in patents with COVID-19.

Terpenoids exist in over 36,000 species (*Augustin et al., 2011*). Terpenoids play a role in the modulation of cellular metabolism, especially in the biosynthesis of sterols and exhibit significant levels of antiviral activity (*Malinowska et* al., 2013). Certain triterpenes have been shown to exhibit effectiveness against HSV1 and HSV2 (*dammarenolic acid, hydroxyhopanone, dammarenediol-II, dammaradienol, ursonic acid, hydroxyoleanonic lactone, hydroxydammarenone-I, shoreic acid and eichlerianic acid*) (*Poehland et al., 1987*).

Essential Oils that Inhibit SARS-CoV-2

Out of a number of essential oils tested for their ability to reduce or eliminate SARS-CoV-2 activity, the main substance in the essential oils was the sesquiterpene hydrocarbon farnesene. The sesquiterpene hydrocarbon farnesene is found in the following essential oils –

Ginger essential oil [3d]

Grapefruit essential oil [3e]

Farnesene is also found in the coatings of Granny Smith Apples the common ant and the codling moth [3f]. When a synthetic form of farnesene was made it the ants it exhibited a provoked rapid attack by aphidicolus ants showing that the ants were responding to an alarm type pheromone. Farnesene is also found hops used to make beer [3g].

Antiviral Essential Oils

Many of the plants that exhibit antiviral activity are aromatic in nature. These include the essential oils of - γ-Terpinene, Limonene, Verbenone, Thymol, Eucalyptol, Chamazulene, Sabinene, trans-Anethole, Caryophyllene, Linalool, Camphenilone, Camphene, Camphor, Borneol, Menthol, Eugenol, Carvacrol, Disulfide, Myrcene, Myrtenol and Verbenone. Also aromatic medicinal plants include Rosmarinus officinalis L., Artemisia annua L., Salvia officinalis L.Pimpinella anisum L and Citrus limon (L.) Osbeck,Eugenia caryophyllata Thunb.

Citrus sp., Curcuma sp., Alpinia galanga, and Caesalpinia sappan
An in-depth study conducted by Utomo and Meiyanto (*2020*) revealed that Citrus sp. showed the highest inhibitory potential against SARS-CoV-2. The next most effective herbs, from best to least were galangal, sappan wood and curcuma [4] [5] [6].

Further Reading
Essential Oils as Antiviral Agents, Potential of Essential Oils to Treat SARS-CoV-2 Infection: An In-Silico Investigation. Joyce Kelly R. da Silva et al. May 2020.

Curcuma longa L. (Zingiberaceae)
Curcumin, the main constituent of the plant species Curcuma longa L. In, has been recommended as a potential clinical option for treating SARS-CoV-2 infection. This is because it exhibits action in several steps of viral infections. These include cellular signaling pathways modulation and protease inhibition, among others (*Zahedipour et al., 2020*)

Using Terpenoids to defeat COVID-19
A recent research study conducted by Shaghaghi (*2020*) looked at the structure of terpinoids and the COVID-19 protease from the databases of PubChem and the Protein Data Bank (PDB). Nine different terpenes were analyzed for their inhibitory effects. Found during this study was thymoquinone, which is extracted from Nigella sativa (black cumin seed). Dynamic computer simulations have shown that thymoquinone interacts with the attachment of SARS-

CoV-2, helping reduce the chance of COVID-19 infection [7] (*Elfiky, 2020*). Hence, it is time to study thymoquinone in clinical trials as a treatment or preventative for COVID-19 (*Ahmad et al., 2020a*).

Additional terpenoids obtained included Bilobalide and Ginkgolide A from Gingko biloba, Salvinorin A derived from Salvia divinorum, citral from Backhousia citriodora, Forscolin from Plectranthus barbatus, Beta Selinene from Apium graveolens, menthol from Mentha and Noscapine extracted from the Papaveraceae family species. The study discovered that terpenoids successfully suppressed virus protease enzyme activity.

HIV Proteases

Certain HIV Proteases may can also be suitable candidates for defeating COVID-19. These include Euphorbia granulate, Ocimum kikim, Acacia nilotica, Ocimum sanctum, Eugenia jambolana, Vitex negundo, Ocimum scharicum and Solanum nigrum. These have been shown to be effective against HIV-reverse transcriptase activity and may show potential for defeating SARS-CoV-2 [7].

Numbered References. Chapter 6

(1) A.D. Sharma, I. Kaur, Molecular docking studies on Jensenone from eucalyptus essential oil as a potential inhibitor of COVID 19 corona virus infection, 2020, doi:10.20944/preprints202003.0455.v1.

(2) S. Ben-Shabat, L. Yarmolinsky, D. Porat, A. Dahan, Antiviral effect of phytochemicals from medicinal plants: Aapplications and drug delivery strategies, Drug Deliv. Transl. Res. 10 (2) (2020) 354-367, doi:10.1007/s13346-019-00691-6.

(3) A.D. Sharma, I. Kaur, Molecular docking studies on Jensenone from eucalyptus essential oil as a potential inhibitor of COVID 19 corona virus infection, 2020, doi:10.20944/preprints202003.0455.v1.

(3a) Geranium and Lemon Essential Oils and Their Active Compounds Downregulate Angiotensin-Converting Enzyme 2 (ACE2), a SARS-CoV-2 Spike Receptor-Binding Domain, in Epithelial Cells. K. J. Senthil Kumar, et al June 2020.

(3b) Promising phytochemicals of traditional Indian herbal steam inhalation therapy to combat COVID-19 - An in silico study. Shanmugaraj Gowrishankar et al. Jan 2021.

(3c) Natural products for COVID-19 prevention and treatment regarding to previous coronavirus infections and novel studies. Motahareh Boozari et al. Sept 2020.

(3d) K.P. Prabhakaran Nair, in The Agronomy and Economy of Turmeric and Ginger, 2013.

(3e) Tzi Bun Ng, ... Jack Ho Wong, in Essential Oils in Food Preservation, Flavor and Safety, 2016.

(3f) Chemistry Of Plant/Insect Interactions. William S. Bowers, in Insect Biology in the Future, 1980.

(3g) Stuart Howe, in The Craft Brewing Handbook, 2020.

(4) M. Akram, et al., Antiviral potential of medicinal plants against HIV, HSV, influenza, hepatitis, and coxsackievirus: a systematic review, Phytother. Res. 32 (5) (2018). 811-822, doi:10.1002/ptr.6024.

(5) M. Wink, Potential of DNA intercalating alkaloids and other plant secondary metabolites against SARS-CoV-2 causing COVID-19, Diversity 12 (5) (2020) 1-10, doi:10.3390/D12050175.

(6) K. Dhama, et al., Medicinal and therapeutic potential of herbs and plant metabolites / extracts countering viral pathogens – current knowledge and future prospects, Curr. Drug Metab. 19 (2018) 3068913, doi:10.2174/1389200219666180129145252.

(7) Mishra et al., 2014; Rege and Chowdhary, 2014; NAIR, 2012; Thayil Seema and Thyagarajan, 2016.

Chapter 7. COVID-19 Resistance Herbs.

PLEASE NOTE - The information in this chapter is for informational purposes only. Some of these substances have not undergone extensive clinical trials, but have been tested by health professionals and medical researchers and have been found to exhibit protective effects or reduce the severity of COVID-19. The majority of the substances in this chapter are natural supplements and herbs.

To date, the United States has the world's 12th-highest percentage of people infected with COVID-19 (*out of 213 countries*). This adds up to approximately 22,484 cases per million or approximately 5.1 times higher than the global average. Contrast this to Japan, which has 657 cases per million.

In a research study titled: *COVID-19: Is There Evidence for the Use of Herbal Medicines as Adjuvant Symptomatic Therapy* that was conducted by Daˆ maris Silveira and colleagues that was published in September 2020, 39 herbal medicines were found to be very likely to appeal to COVID-19 patients, with the benefits/risks assessment of the herbs being positive in 5 cases.

Five herbs were found as potentially good candidates in helping mitigate early or mild symptoms of flu, cold and bronchitis (in the context of COVID-19). These plants were Glycyrrhiza glabra, Hedera helix, Althaea officinalis, Commiphora molmol and Sambucus nigra. These herbs exhibit safety margins which are superior to those of reference drugs; with enough merit as to recommend them for clinical use as adjuvants in treating early/mild cases of COVID-19.

A second group of herbs considered as promising candidates consisted of the following - Echinacea angustifolia, Echinacea purpurea, Eucalyptus globulus essential oil, Allium sativum, Andrographis paniculata, Justicia pectoralis, Magnolia officinalis, Mikania glomerata Pelargonium sidoides, Zingiber officinale, Pimpinella anisum and Salix sp.

The authors in the study recommended that the scientific community prioritize these herbs into full integration into clinical use, due to the fact that the three reference drugs currently in use for target symptoms may help to mitigate the discomfort in early stages of COVID-19 due to their immunomodulatory, antitussive and anti-inflammatory properties.

Persian herbs
The Persian herbs Allium sativum, Cerasus avium, Rubia tinctorum, Berberis integerrima, Alcea digitata and Peganum harmala have been recommended for COVID-19 prevention after proper evaluation (*Hiedary et al., 2020*).

A. sativum has been shown to impede the viral replication of SARS-CoV (*Nourazarian et al., 2016; Keyaerts et al., 2007*).

Herbs and Herbal Formulas Scientifically Proven to Disrupt and Destroy Bad Viruses

Piper Betel
Sengupta (*2019*) found that Piper Betel contained Aurantiamide, which was shown to inhibit Coronavirus. Piper Betel also contains piperol, chavibetol, eugenol, catechol, caryophyllene, etragol, betlol and shiwh help support the body's defenses by reducing infection (*Sengupta, 2019*). Apart from aurantiamide, other potential

peptide that has role in combating COVID-19 is peptide EK1 (*Lu et al., 2020c*).

A. paniculata
Liu et al. (*2020a*) showed A. paniculata repressed SARS-CoV and SARS-CoV-2 pathogenesis.

Herbs that specifically attack SARS-CoV-2
Houttuynia cordata
This herb has shown effectiveness against SARS-CoV through inhibition of 3CL-proteases and RNA-polymerases (*Yu et al., 2012*) and Cynara scolymus, Hyoscyamus niger, Verbascum thapsus and Justicia adhatoda have been shown to attack SARS-CoV-2 as well as influenza virus and also inhinit Ca2+ channels (*Gilani et al., 2008*).

Sambucus ebulus
Sambucus ebulus has been shown to attack enveloped viruses (*Ganjhu et al., 2015*).

25-hydroxy-cholesterol
25-hydroxy-cholesterol shows broad antiviral activity. It works by blocking membrane fusion in the viral infection stage [1].

Dihydrotanshinone
Dihydrotanshinone was shown to both block viral entry possibly inhibit the replication of bad viruses [2].

A list of Plants Screened for their effectiveness against COVID-19
More than 200 plant extracts against two SARS-CoV viral strains (BJ-001 and BJ-006) were screened. The study revealed that an ethanol cortex extract of Lycorisradiata

(Amaryllidaceae) inhibited both strains (EC50 2.4 and 2.1 µM, respectively). The antiviral activity was tributed to the alkaloid fraction lycorine [3].

Further Reading
Ma et al. reported that the Liu-Shen formula exhibited favorable inhibitory effects against SARS-CoV-2 replication as well as virus-induced inflammation (in vitro) most likely via suppressing NF-κB pathways (Ma et al., 2020).

Natural and Nature-Derived Products Targeting Human Coronaviruses. Konstantina Vougogiannopoulou et al. Jan 2021. Department of Pharmacognosy and Natural Products Chemistry, Faculty of Pharmacy, National and Kapodistrian University of Athens, Panepistimiopolis Zografou, 15771 Athens, Greece.

Numbered References. Chapter 7

(1) Wang, S.; Li, W.; Hui, H.; Tiwari, S.K.; Zhang, Q.; Croker, B.A.; Rawlings, S.; Smith, D.; Carlin, A.F.; Rana, T.M. Cholesterol 25-Hydroxylase inhibits SARS-CoV-2 and other coronaviruses by depleting membrane cholesterol. EMBO J. 2020.

(2) Kim, J.Y.; Kim, Y., II; Park, S.J.; Kim, L.K.; Choi, Y.K.; Kim, S.-H. Safe, high-throughput screening of natural compounds of MERS-CoV entry inhibitors using a pseudovirus expressing MERS-CoV spike protein. Int. J.Antimicrob. Agents 2018, 52, 730–732.

(3) Li, S.-Y.; Chen, C.; Zhang, H.-Q.; Guo, H.-Y.; Wang, H.; Wang, L.; Zhang, X.; Hua, S.-N.; Yu, J.; Xiao, P.-G. Identification of natural compounds with antiviral activities against SARS-associated coronavirus. Antivir. Res. 2005, 67, 18–23.

Chapter 8. Chinese Herbal Tablets, Capsules and Polyphenols.

My personal COVID-19 Resistance Formula
First I would like to share the formula that I use. I have found from my own personal experience during the last 9 months that using this formula before going into a populated area or when returning from a populated area works well for me. It uses the herb Ajwain (*Trachyspermum ammi L*) which has been shown to protect DNA [1]. All healing begins when the DNA of the body is in healthy shape.

The Formula is as follows -
Add the below extracts to 1/2 cup of water -

5 Drops of St. Germain Extract.
10 Drops of Ajwain Extract

Drink and take with the following supplements -

1 to 1 1/2 selenium tablets
2 Cod Liver Oil Capsules (Vitamin D)
1 Vitamin D3 Capsule

A formula to Strengthen The Lungs
A study conducted on rats showed that an ethanol extract Black Cumin Seed (1:4) and chopped seeds exhibited ameliorating effects on oxidative stress and lung inflammation COVID-19 [1b].

1 cup of Apple Juice with 4 to 6 drops of Rhodioa Rosea extract added.

Substances in Rhodiola rosea may promote nerve regeneration

Salidriside, a phenylpropanoid glycoside, is abundant in Rhodiola rosea. Salidriside has been shown in many studies to exhibit neuroprotective effects, making it a promising agent for nerve recovery. For example, studies by Sheng QS et al. stated Salidriside achieved successful nerve regeneration in experiments on rats, evidenced by walking track analysis [2]. In a recent study published in 2017, in just 12 weeks nerve regeneration was witnessed in studies conducted on rats that had nerve injuries when given a combination of Salidriside and lactic-co-glycolic acid. The study concluded that Salidriside may provide re-engineered nerves for regeneration of myelinated nerve fibers [3].

Further Reading
Zhang, J. K. et al. Protection by salidroside against bone loss via inhibition of oxidative stress and bone-resorbing mediators. (2013).

Echinacea

Echinacea's unique gift is that it has the ability to penetrate the membranes of bad viruses. This may make it a promising treatment for COVID-19 [4].

Echinacea has been shown to reduce influenza infection in mice [5].

A research study discovered that a particular type of Echinacea inhibited specific coronaviruses which included (HCoV) 229E, MERS and SARS-CoVs. Researchers stated it could potentially have similar effects on SARS-CoV-2, the coronavirus that causes COVID-19, although it was not tested at the time the study was published.

Echinacea synergizes with garlic, ginseng, licorace herb, black seed, curcumin, vigamin D, vitamin C and zinc.

Hence you may find these substances in some commercial preparations that sell Echinacea.

Echinacea Recommended Dosages

Echinacea is recommended to be taken no more than 10 days in a row in order to avoid an over reactive immune system. The World Health Organization states to take Echinacea a maximum of 8 weeks at daily doses of between 80 and 1,500 daily. Echinacea should be avoided if one is pregnant or nursing [6].

Another immune system booster is copper. Copper (in trace element form) has shown to help enhance the immune system (Li et al., 2019).

Further Reading

Can Echinacea be a potential candidate to target immunity, inflammation and infection - The trinity of coronavirus disease 2019. Nagoor Meeran et al. 2021.

Echinacea—A Source of Potent Antivirals for Respiratory Virus Infections. James Hudson and Selvarani Vimalanathan. July 2011.

Supplements for COVID-19: A modifiable environmental risk. Trevor K. Younga and John G. Zampella. May 2020.

Traditional Herbal Medicine Candidates as Complementary Treatments for COVID-19: A Review of Their Mechanisms, Pros and Cons. Rhea Veda Nugraha et al. Oct 2020.

Bee Propolis

Bee Propolis is commonly used to treat advanced forms of cancer. Anticancer constituents present in propolis depend upon the region and harvesting properties. For instance, the anti-cancer element in Brazilian propolis is called Artepillin C (ARC). However in the sub-tropical regions of Okinawa Japan and Taiwan it is the polyphenols in bee propolis that have stronger anti-cancer effects [7]. Hence, where the Bee Propolis is obtained from will determine its effectiveness when used for medicinal purposes. One of the most powerful forms of Bee Propolis is a CAPE-containing propolis known as 'Bio 30'. This type of Bee Propolis is produced in New Zealand (*Maruta, 2014*).

Polyphenols for Defeating COVID-19

Natural polyphenols have been shown to be potent inhibitors of COVID-19 in a study conducted by Adem et al. (2020). In his research study, the effectiveness of herbal plants was based on their bioactive constituent's versus flavonoids. They were analyzed for their effectiveness against the COVID-19 virus by docking techniques. The COVID-19 virus was than docked with 80 various flavonoids. The study found that compounds such as diosmin, rutin, apiin, hesperidin and diacetylcurcumin might play a major role in allievating the symptoms of patients diagnosed with COVID-19.

Research studies by Wink showed that polyphenols bind easily with lipoproteins of a virus' envelope. This binding activity helps prevent the virus from entering the cells and causing devastation [8].

Quercetin

I have written extensively in my series of anti-aging books, that Quercetin is one of the most potent substances that reverses aging due to its abundance of polyphenols. Studies by Boyu Pan et, al. found that quercetin has a receptor blocking effect as well as a virus-neutralizing effect on SARS-CoV-2. This makes it a promising candidate against COVID-19 [8a].

A research study titled: *The effect of quercetin on the prevention or treatment of COVID-19 and other respiratory tract infections in humans* that was conducted by Monique Aucoin and colleagues and published in July of 2020 stated the following -

"*One study reported a decrease in the incidence of upper respiratory tract infections following a competitive athletic event. A larger clinical trial reported a benefit in older athletic adults.*"

The Herbal Composition called Gene-Eden-VIR/Novirin
Gene-Eden-VIR/Novirin has shown to be effective against numerous viruses. The mixture is composed of quercetin, green tea, licorice herb, cinnamon and selenium (*Polansky and Lori, 2020*). A recent 2020 study found it disrupted viral entry, replication, viral proteases and infection which enhanced the immune system against SARS-CoV-2 respectively (*Polansky and Lori, 2020*).

Cinnamon
A study by Zuang et al. demonstrated that an extract of cinnamon inhibited wild-type SARS-CoV (in vitro) with an IC50 of 43 µM [8b].

Sang Ju Yin plus Yu Ping Feng San Protects High Risk Workers from SARS
Lau and colleagues stated during the SARS outbreak, 1063 volunteers, which included 926 hospital workers and 37

laboratory technicians that worked in high-risk virus labs took a TCM herbal extract called Sang Ju Yin plus Yu Ping Feng San. The study found that compared with the 0.4% of infection in the control group, none of TCM users became infected. Also there was some evidence that Sang Ju Yin plus Yu Ping Feng San may modulate the body's T cells. When the Sang Ju Yin plus Yu Ping Feng San formula was tested in a controlled clinical study, it shortened the disease course and resulted in a marked improvement of symptoms [8c].

Astragalus
In China, astragalus, alone or in combination in with other herbs has been suggested to potentially help prevent COVID-19 infections [9].

Astragalus also has anti-inflammatory and anti-viral effects. This includes resistance activity against a particular type of coronavirus that commonly infects poultry (*Jin, Int J Biol Macromol 2014; Zhang, Microb Pathog 2018*). Now let's move onto looking at Chinese Herbal Tablets and Capsules.

Astragalus in detail
Astragalus membranaceus exhibits a wide variety of pharmacological effects. These include regulating the body's immune function and antiviral activity. Astragalus is widely in TCM clinical practice due to its significant curative effects. It also enhances the body's respiratory immune system and regulates the secretion of mucous in the body's respiratory tract (*Qin et al., 2017*).

Astragalus membranaceus also increases the body's white blood cells and promotes cellular immunity as well as humoral immunity. This is what makes it responsible for enhancing the body's immune system. Studies have found that Astragalus membranaceus reduced inflammation, enhanced the body's resistance to viruses and played various roles responsible for protecting the body against broad-spectrum antiviral hazards (*Wang et al., 2017*).

Traditional Chinese Medicine Herbs (TCM) used for the treatment of COVID-19. Case Reviews and Recent Studies.

How does Traditional Chinese Medicine (TCM) Work?
TCM methods and herbs used for neutralizing infections from epidemics is based upon the theory of restoring balance to the human immune system. This in turn naturally ends up defeating the viral infection. Most TCM herbal preparations aim at targeting the lung meridian, which connects the body's lung and large intestine regions. The interconnection between the lung (including the body's upper respiratory system) and the body's intestine explain why specific TCM herbal formulas exhibited powerful healing effects upon the patients' lungs (by relieving congestion) and the relief of stomach diarrhea, which are dual characteristics of COVID-19 infection. In simple summary, the primary mainstream theory of treating COVID-19 patients is by using the proper herbal preparations which will expel toxic moisture from the upper respiratory regions of the body and improve and clear intestinal obstructions [10].

Please Note - Some herbs used in TCM (*Traditional Chinese Medicine*) can mimic, magnify, or sometimes oppose the effect of conventional pharmaceutical medications. Also SARS-CoV-2 is the coronavirus that causes COVID-19.

The Qing Fei Pai Du Tang Formula
In a report titled: *Administration of Traditional Chinese Medicine* published February 5th, 2020, 214 COVID-19 patients were treated with Qing Fei Pai Du Tang in Shanxi,

Hebei, Heilongjiang and Shaanxi Provinces with an overall success rate of ≥ 90%. The symptoms of the majority of patients (≥60%) were improved, and the illness of others (30%) was stabilized [11].

In addition, 701 COVID-19 patients were treated with the Qing Fei Pai Du Tang formula in 10 Chinese provinces in China. The research stated that 130 patients (18.5%) were completely cured after treatment with the formula [11a].

The Qing Fei Pai Du Tang Formula
In addition, 701 COVID-19 patients were given Qing Fei Pai Du Tang in 10 provinces in China. Out of this group, 130 patients (18.5%) were completely cured after treatment. This simple herbal treatment resulted in the full disappearance of the symptoms of COVID-19 such as fever and cough in 51 of the patients tested (7.27%). Also improvement took place in 268 of the patients (38.2%) and in 212 of the patients (30.2%) [12].

The Lian Hua Qing Wen Capsule Formula
The Lian Hua Qing Wen Capsule exhibited the ability to inhibit various influenza viruses. It was reported to block early stages of infection caused by the influenza virus as well as inhibit the virus-induced gene expression of IL-6, IL-8, IP-10, TNF-a and MCP-1 [12a].

Studies by Yao, et al. and Lu, et al. analyzed the clinical effectiveness of a formula called Lian Hua Qing Wen in Capsule form administered to COVID-19 patients. The study found the herbs relieved major symptoms such as cough and fever and it showed remarkable potential to promote recovery [13] [14].

Additional COVID-19 Herbal Formulas
Shu Feng Jie Du Capsule

Huo Xiang Zheng Qi Shui
Lian Hua Qing Wen Capsule and Jin Hua Qing Gan Granule

Herbal formulas for critical patients with COVID-19 [15]

Sheng Mai Injection
Shen Fu Injection
Su He Xiang Pill
An Gong Niu Huang Pill
Xue Bi Jing Injection
Re Du Ning Injection
Tan Re Qing Injection/
Su He Xiang Pill

The 10 most Commonly used Herbs used to Treat COVID-19
In a meta-analysis of the most used herbs to treat COVID-19 administered in 23 Chinese provinces [16] by, Luo, et al., the most frequent herbs were as follows -

Astragalus membranaceus
Glycyrrhizae uralensis
Atractylodis Rhizoma
Radix platycodonis
Agastache rugosa
Saposhnikoviae divaricata
Rhizoma Atractylodis Macrocephalae
Lonicerae Japonicae Flos
Fructus forsythia and Cyrtomium fortune

A study conducted by Xu, et al. [17] discovered that a combination of Astragalus and Yu Ping Feng were utilized in 13 prevention programs for "reinforcing vital qi". In TCM this terminology describes a return to balance of the human immune system.

The Sang Ju Yin plus Yu Ping Feng San Extract

This formula has been attributed to reducing the number of deaths gradually from 4% to 1% after May 20th 2003 during the SARS outbreak [18]. The researchers discovered to their surprise that compared to 0.4% of people infected, compared to the control group, none of the users of the formula became infected. The study goes on to state that evidence exists that the Sang Ju Yin plus Yu Ping Feng San formula modulates the body's natural T cells, which are cells that enhance the immune system [19].

Herbs Scientifically Proven for enhancing Lung Strength and Oxygen Capacity

The Lian Hua Qing Wen Capsule Formula

A research study conducted by Dong et al. stated that patients diagnosed with chronic obstructive pulmonary disease who took Lian Hua Qing Wen Capsules reported levels of their IL-17, IL-8, TNF-α and IL-23 in the sputum and of IL-8 and IL-17 in their blood was markedly decreased. The IL series is a method of specific actions that take place to protect the body from disease such as from pathogens or to restore balance to the immune system [20].

Traditional Chinese Medicine Herbs used for Treating Inflammation

Many people who died from SARS and COVID-19 have been found to exhibit extreme inflammation. Hence, anti-inflammatory herbs may be of benefit in reducing the severity of this disease [21].

The Shuang Huang Lian Formula

Shuang Huang Lian is a herbal combination made from Scutellariae radix, Lonicerae japonicae Flos and Fructus

Forsythiae. It has been shown to inhibit SARS-CoV-2. The study also discovered that the herbal combination significantly reduced inflammation [22] [23].

Scutellariae radix in detail
Scutellariae radix is the root of Scutellaria baicalensis Georgi. This plant is used for fire purging, heat clearing, detoxification and homeostasis. Scutellariae radix's antiviral, anti-tumour, anti-microbial and anti-inflammatory effects have been well documented [23a].

The Dang Gui Long Hui Pill Formula
The substance Indirubin can be found in a herbal formula called Dang Gui Long Hui Pill, which has been found to exhibit powerful antiviral and immunomodulatory properties [24].

The Sang Ju Yin and Yu Ping Feng San Formulas
A research study by Poon et al. demonstrated that the administration of the formulas Sang Ju Yin and Yu Ping Feng San exerted powerful immunomodulatory effects that help prevent viral infections including SARS-CoV [25] [26].

C. ineme
C. ineme was observed to reduce virus activity (*Nourazarian et al., 2016; Keyaerts et al., 2007*).

Numbered References. Chapter 8

(1) Assessment of free radical scavenging potential and oxidative DNA damage preventive activity of Trachyspermum ammi L. (carom) and Foeniculum vulgare Mill. (fennel) seed extracts.

(1b) Is There Evidence for the Use of Herbal Medicines as Adjuvant Symptomatic Therapy? Daˆ maris Silveira et al. September 2020).

(2) Sheng, Q. S., Wang, Z. J., Zhang, J. & Zhang, Y. G. Salidroside promotes peripheral nerve regeneration following crush injury to the sciatic nerve in rats (2013).

(3) Salidroside promotes peripheral nerve regeneration based on tissue engineering strategy using Schwann cells and PLGA: in vitro and in vivo. Hui Liu et al. Jan 2017.

(4) M. Sharma, S. A. Anderson, R. Schoop, and J. B. Hudson, "Induction of multiple pro-inflammatory cytokines by respiratory viruses and reversal by standardized Echinacea, a potent antiviral herbal extract," Antiviral Research, vol. 83, no. 2, pp. 165–170, 2009.

(5) Can Echinacea be a potential candidate to target immunity, inflmmation and infection - The trinity of coronavirus disease 2019. Nagoor Meeran et al. 2021.

(6) The effect of Echinacea spp. on the prevention or treatment of COVID-19 and other respiratory tract infections in humans: A rapid review.

(7) Herbal immune-boosters: Substantial warriors of pandemic Covid-19 battle. Kanika Khannaa et al. Sept 2020.

(8) M. Wink, Potential of DNA intercalating alkaloids and other plant secondary metabolites against SARS-CoV-2 causing COVID-19, Diversity 12 (5) (2020) 1-10, doi:10.3390/D12050175.

(8a) (8a) B. Pan, S. Fang, J. Zhang, Y. Pan, H. Liu, Y. Wang, M. Li, L. Liu, Chinese herbal compounds against SARS-CoV-2: puerarin and quercetin impair the binding of viral S-protein to ACE2 receptor, Comput. Struct. Biotechnol. J. 18 (2020) 3518-3527.

(8b) Traditional Chinese Medicine in the Treatment of Patients Infected with 2019-New Coronavirus (SARS-CoV-2): A Review and Perspective. Yang Yang et al. March 2020.

(8c) Zhuang M, Jiang H, Suzuki Y, Li X, Xiao P, Tanaka T, et al. Procyanidins and butanol extract of Cinnamomi cortex inhibit SARS-CoV infection. Antiviral Res. 2009;82:73-81. doi:10.1016/j.antiviral.2009.02.001.

(9) Traditional Chinese Medicine in the Treatment of Patients Infected with 2019-New Coronavirus (SARS-CoV-2): A Review and Perspective. Yang Yang et al. 2020.

(10) Traditional Chinese herbal medicine at the forefront battle against COVID19: Clinical experience and scientific basis. David Y.W. Lee et al. Sept 2020.

(11) Zhao J, Tian SS, Yang J, Liu J, Zhang WD. Investigating the mechanism of Qing-Fei-Pai-Du-Tang for the treatment of Novel Coronavirus Pneumonia by network pharmacology. Chin Herb Med. 2020. pp. 1-7.

(11a) Traditional Chinese Medicine in the Treatment of Patients Infected with 2019 - New Coronavirus (SARS-CoV-2): A Review and Perspective. Yang Yang and Md Sahidul Islam. March 2020.

(12) National Health Commission of the People's Republic of China. Transcript of press conference in 17, February, 2020.

http://www.nhc.gov.cn/xcs/s3574/202002/f12a62d10c2a48c6895cedf2faea6e1f. shtml. 2020.

(12a) Ding Y, Zeng L, Li R, Chen Q, Zhou B, Chen Q, et al. The Chinese prescription lianhuaqingwen capsule exerts anti-influenza activity through the inhibition of viral propagation and impacts immune function. BMC Complement Altern Med. 2017; 17: 130.

(13) Yao KT, Liu MY, Li X, Huang JH, Cai HB. Retrospective Clinical Analysis on Treatment of Novel Coronavirus-infected Pneumonia with Traditional Chinese Medicine Lianhua Qingwen. Chin J Exp Tradit Med Form. 2020. pp. 1-7.

(14) Lv RB, Wang WJ, Li X. Treatment of suspected new coronavirus pneumonia with Chinese medicine Lianhua Qingwen Clinical observation of 63 suspected cases. J Tradit Chin Med. 2020. pp. 1-5.

(15) Traditional Chinese Medicine in the Treatment of Patients Infected with 2019-New Coronavirus (SARS-CoV-2): A Review and Perspective. Yang Yang et al. 2020.

(16) Luo H, Tang QL, Shang YX, Liang SB, Yang M, Robinson N, Can Chinese Medicine Be Used for Prevention of Corona Virus Disease 2019 (COVID-19)? A Review of Historical Classics, Research Evidence and Current Prevention Programs. Chin J Integr Med. 2020.

(17) Xu X, Zhang Y, Li X, Li XX. Analysis on prevention plan of corona virus disease-19 (COVID-19) by traditional Chinese medicine in various regions. Chin Herb Med. 2020. pp. 1-7.

(18) T.F. Lau, Leung PC, Wong ELY, Fong C, Cheng KF, Zhang SC, et al. Using Herbal Medicine as a Means of Prevention Experience During the SARS Crisis. Am J Chin Med. 2005;33:345-56.

(19) Poon PM, Wong CK, Fung KP, Fong CY, Wong EL, Lau JT. et al. Immunomodulatory effects of a traditional Chinese medicine with potential antiviral activity: a self-control study. Am J Chin Med. 2006;34:13-21.

(20) Arabi YM, Mandourah Y, Al-Hameed F, Sindi AA, Almekhlafi GA, Hussein MA. et al. Corticosteroid Therapy for Critically Ill Patients with Middle East Respiratory Syndrome. Am J Respir Crit Care Med. 2018;197:757-67.

(21) Lu H. Drug treatment options for the 2019-new coronavirus (2019-nCoV) Biosci Trends. 2020.

(22) Science CAo. Researchers in Shanghai Institute of Drugs and Wuhan Virus Institute discovered that the Chinese patent medicine Shuanghuanglian oral liquid can inhibit the 2019-new coronavirus.; 2020.

(23) Gao Y, Fang L, Cai R, Zong C, Chen X, Lu J. et al. Shuang-Huang-Lian exerts anti-inflammatory and anti-oxidative activities in lipopolysaccharide-stimulated murine alveolar macrophages. Phytomedicine. 2014;21:461-9.

(23a) Wang ZL, Wang S, Kuang Y, et al. A comprehensive review on phytochemistry, pharmacology, and flavonoid biosynthesis of Scutellaria baicalensis. Pharm Biol 2018;56:465-84.

(24) Chan MC, Chan RW, Mok CK, Mak NK, Wong RN. Indirubin-3'-oxime as an antiviral and immunomodulatory agent in treatment of severe human influenza virus infection. Hong Kong Med J. 2018;24(Suppl 6):45-7.

(25) Poon PM, Wong CK, Fung KP, Fong CY, Wong EL, Lau JT. et al. Immunomodulatory effects of a traditional Chinese medicine with potential antiviral activity: a self-control study. Am J Chin Med. 2006;34:13-21.

(26) Li S, Chen C, Zhang H, Guo H, Wang H, Wang L. et al. Identification of natural compounds with antiviral activities against SARS-associated coronavirus. Antiviral Res. 2005;67:18–23.

Chapter 9. Herbs and Plants Scientifically Proven to Treat Fever, Cough, Asthma, Chronic bronchitis and the Common Cold.

These herbs have been mentioned in the research study titled: COVID-19: *Is There Evidence for the Use of Herbal Medicines as Adjuvant Symptomatic Therapy* that was conducted by Daˆ maris Silveira and colleagues that was published in September 2020. The herbs were mentioned as potentially good candidates in helping mitigate early or mild symptoms of flu, cold and bronchitis (in the context of COVID-19).

Hedera helix L. - Araliaceae (Leaves)
This herb is used for coughs and respiratory diseases (*Hong et al., 2015; Pizzorno et al., 2016*). It has also found use in relieving asthma, acute and chronic bronchitis and pneumonia (*Hong et al., 2015; Pizzorno et al., 2016*). Araliaceae has been subjected to a clinical trial for its effectiveness against bronchial asthma and the improvement of airway resistance (*Hofmann et al., 2003; Guo et al., 2006; Holzinger and Chenot, 2011*).

Justicia pectoralis Jacq. (Jacq.)- Acanthaceae (Leaves)
Justicia pectoralis is used for the treatment of asthma. An extract of Justicia pectoralis was shown to inhibit the tracheal muscles of rats with asthma, showing it exhibits anti-asthma potential (*Moura et al., 2017*). In another study, an extract of J. pectoralis reduced the formation of histamine-induced wheals in guinea pigs and also reduced histamine-induced tracheal smooth muscle contractions

(*Cameron et al., 2015*) making it a powerful natural plant herb for helping treat asthma.

Further Reading
Identification of alkaloids from Justicia adhatoda as potent SARS CoV-2 main protease inhibitors: An in silico perspective. Rajesh Ghosh et al. Oct 2020.

Magnolia officinalis Rehder & E.H. Wilson - Magnoliaceae (Bark)
Magnolia officinalis has been scientifically proven to help treat asthma. Honokiol (an anti-aging substance) and Magnolol are the main ingredients of magnolia bark. Animal studies demonstrated multiple properties of honokiol; including anti-asthma properties (through IL4 and IFN-NF-kB) (*Hong et al., 2018*). It also exhibits antihistamine properties (*Shin et al., 2001*) as well as anti-HIV (human immunodeficiency viruses) properties (*Amblard et al., 2006*). A clinical trial involving preparations of Magnolia showed it was beneficial for treating asthma as well as oral health (*Campus et al., 2011*). In another research study involving 148 patients with mild to moderate asthma given an extract of Magnoliae, the patients exhibited reduced complications regarding their asthma (*Park et al.,2012*).

Recommended Dosage
A dose of 750 mg per person daily (approximately 15 and 60 mg/person per day of honokiol and magnolol respectively) is recommended (*Garrison and Chambliss,2006*).

Mikania glomerata Spreng and M. laevigata Sch.Bip. ex Baker Asteraceae (Leaves)
Mikania glomerata is used in Brazil for cough, asthma and throat inflammation (*Agra et al., 2008; Brandao et al., 2009), (BRASIL, 2011; BRASIL, 2017; BRASIL, 2018*). An extract of Mikania glomerata Spreng was shown to reduce the contractile effect of histamine in guinea-pigs and human bronchi (*Moura et al., 2002*). Also a fraction of M. glomerata extract resulted in the inhibition of leukocyte infiltration in studies done on rats (*Fierro et al., 1999*).

Chemical composition - terpenoids and steroids (e.g., friedelin, ent-kaurenoic acid, ent-kaur-16(17)-en-19-oic acid, ent-beyer-15(16)-en-19-oic acid, ent-15b-benzoyloxykaur16(17)- en-19-oic acid and grandifloric acid. Essential oil (germacrene D and b-caryophyllene as the major components) (*Ueno and Sawaya, 2019*); coumarins, phenolic acids (chlorogenic and caffeoylquinic acids) (*Lazzari Almeida et al., 2017*); ent-cinnamoylgrandifloric acid, ent-benzoylgrandifloric acid ,17-hydroxy-ent-kaur-15(16)-en-19-oic acid, stigmasterol, b-sitosterol) (*Veneziani and Oliveira, 1999; Bertolucci et al., 2013*).

Recommended Dosage
3 g of dried leaves in 150 ml; used as an infusion. Taken twice daily.

Ocimum gratissimum L. -Lamiaceae (Leaves)
Ocimum gratisssimum is used to treat influenza, fever, asthma, cold and bronchitis (*WHO, 2002*). An aqueous extract of O. gratissimum was shown in guinea-pigs to exhibit anti-asthma properties. It also reduced the number of cough episodes 80% (*Ozolua et al., 2016*). In another study an essential oil of O. gratissimum exhibited antinociceptive effects in studies done on mice (*Rabelo et

al., 2003; Paula-Freire et al., 2013). Also a flavonoid-rich fraction of O. gratissimum was shown to exhibit anti-inflammatory effects, causing a reduction in the number of the leucocytes in the peritoneum. It also inhibited COX-2 and iNOS (in the same manner than indomethacin) and inhibited LPS-induced TNF-a production and NO, IL-1b in RAW 264.7 cells (Ajayi et al., 2017).

Chemical composition. Essential oil (eugenol, thymol, and 1,8-cineol as the major components) (Prabhu et al., 2009; Monga et al., 2017); triterpenes (ursolic acid) (Prabhu et al., 2009; BRASIL, 2015b; Siva et al., 2016; Monga et al., 2017), phenolics (quercetin and derivatives, luteolin and derivatives, kaempferol and derivatives, catechin, epi-catechin, cafeic acid).

Recommended Dosage
1-3 g placed in 150 ml of boiling water; used as an infusion. Taken three to four times a day (BRASIL, 2019b).

Pelargonium sidoides DC and/or Pelargonium reniforme Curt. -Geraniaceae (Root)
Pelargonium sidoides is used to treat the common cold (EMA, 2018c), bronchitis and coughing (COLOMBIA, 2008). Umkaloabo preparations can be bought in certain European Countries where it is widely used to treat acute bronchitis and other respiratory conditions (EMA, 2018c).

Pelargonium sidoides has been tested in clinical settings for coughs. A study involving 124 adults diagnosed with acute bronchitis consumed 30 drops of EPs 7630®, for a total of seven days. The participants in the study exhibited a significant improvement regarding the Bronchitis Severity Score (BSS) compared with a placebo group (Chuchalin et al., 2005). A Cochrane review stated that P. sidoides might be helpful in helping alleviate the common cold and persons with acute rhinosinusitis may also benefit from taking P. sidoides (*Timmer et al., 2013*).

Pimpinella anisum L. – Apiaceae (Fruits)
Pimpinella anisum is used for fevers and coughing (*WHO, 2009; CHILE, 2010*) as well as an antispasmodic (*WHO, 2009; CHILE, 2010; BRASIL, 2011*). A research study examined the bronchodilator activity of P. anisum in 50 patients with bronchial asthma. The participant's took the herb as tea (2 g in 200 ml of water) twice daily for a total of 40 days. All the participants in the study exhibited a reduction of coughing after 2 weeks (going from 6 + episodes/day to none). It was also noted that the participant's exhibited an improvement in the ability to hold their breath as well as respiratory rate (*Paheerathan, 2019*). Other studies found that ethanol and aqueous extracts of P. anisum exhibited myorelaxant effects in the tracheal chains of guinea-pigs. The effect was similar to theophylline. However, the essential oil did not exhibit a significant effect (*Boskabady and RamazaniAssari, 2001*), which could have been due to the quality of the essential oil or other factors. Overall this herb is highly recommended for treating asthma-related cough.

Chemical composition –
Essential oil (trans-anethole as the main component (*Orav et al., 2008*); chlorogenic acid derivatives; flavonoids (orientin, vitexin and coumarin – also anti-aging substances); triterpenes and steroidal compounds (*Zobel et al., 1991; Reichling and Galati, 2004; Abdollahi Fard, 2012*).

Recommended Dosage
1,5 g of the dried fruits placed in 150 ml of boiling water. Used as an infusion. Taken up to three times daily (*BRASIL, 2011; Barnes et al., 2012; EMA, 2013b*).

Platycodon chinensis (Jacq). A.DC. [syn. Platycodon grandiflorus (Jacq.) A.DC.] – Campanulaceae (Roots)
Platycodon is used for coughing (*WHO, 1999*) as an expectorant (*WHO, 1999*) and for sore throat and related infections (*PRC, 1992; Li Y. H. et al., 2013*). It contains 2% Triterpene saponins.

Platycodon chinensis has been experimentally proven in studies to relieve coughing and fever in mice (*Oh et al., 2010; Zhang et al., 2015*). An aqueous extract of P. chinensis demonstrated anti-inflammatory activity in a study on rats The extract also inhibited the production of cytokines as well as the expression of COX-2 (*Kim et al., 2006*).

Polypodium vulgare L. – Polypodiaceae (Rhizomes)
Polypodium vulgare is used for coughing as well as related respiratory diseases. A hydroalcoholic extract of Polypodiu vulgare was shown to exhibit a myorelaxant dose-dependent effect in rabbits' isolated tracheal preparation. The effect was cholinergic-like (*Naz et al., 2016*). Studies have stated that the antitussive and expectorant effects of saponins exhibit benefical effects (*Hostettmann and Marston, 2005*) and that saponins (in fresh plants) exhibit cough reducing properties (*Høeg, 1984*).

Chemical composition -
Flavonoids (*Grzybek, 1976; Karl et al.,1982*); triterpenes (*Devys et al., 1969; Robinson et al., 1973; EMA, 2008b*); phytoecdysteroids (*Arai et al., 1991; Yamada et al., 1992; Marco et al., 1993; Coll et al., 1994; Reixach et al., 1996; Messeguer et al., 1998; Simon et al., 2011*); hydroxycinnamic

acids (caffeic acid 4'-glucoside, 0.6% in the rhizome) (*Jizba and Herout, 1967; Grzybek, 1976*).

Recommended Dosage
4-5 g, taken as decoction three to four times daily. Not to be used for more than 7 days in a row (*EMA, 2008c*).

Salix alba L., Salix sp. - Salicaceae (Cortex)
Salix alba is as antipyretic (*BRASIL, 2011; EMA, 2017d*) and it exhibits anti-inflammatory effects. It is used for treating the common cold and flu (*WHO, 2009*). Salix alba has been proven in studies to reduce fever as well as exhibit significant analgesic effects. It also exhibits anti-inflammatory properties in studies on mice. Most important, it has shown more potency than the drug aspirin in all doses reviewed and tested (*Gyawali et al., 2013*). A randomized study involving 210 patients with low back pain took the bark extract with 120 mg or 240 mg of salicin or a placebo over the course of a month. During the final week of treatment, 39% of the patients stated they were free of pain (in the highest doses) and 21% stated their pain was gone for the low doses; with 6% stating their pain was gone for the placebo group (*Chrubasik et al., 2000*).

Zingiber officinale Roscoe - Zingiberaceae (Rhizome)
Also known as Ginger. Zingiber officinale is used for treating coughs and colds (*COLOMBIA, 2008*). It also is used to relieve asthma (*WHO, 1999*) and as an expectorant (BRASIL, 2011). Studies have found Zingiber officinale is beneficial for reducing fever (*Ueki et al., 2008; Akbar, 2020*) and it also exhibits antipyretic, analgesic and anti-inflammatory, properties (*Mascolo et al., 1989; El-Abhar et al., 2008; Sepahvand et al., 2010; Ahmed et al., 2011; Darvishzadeh-Mahani et al., 2012; Hsiang et al., 2013; Rashidian et al., 2014*). The anti-inflammatory effects are

well documented in vivo as well as in vitro models (*Thomson et al., 2002; Ali et al., 2008), (Rehman et al., 2011)*. Moreover the 6-gingerol and 6-shogaol found in Zingiber officinale exhibits anti-platelet aggregation activity in vitro (*Liao et al., 2012*).

In a research study involving 32 patients diagnosed with acute respiratory distress syndrome (ARDS), the patients received an enteral diet that was enriched with ginger for a total of 21 days. On the fifth day, the patients exhibited lower serum levels of IL-1, IL6, and TNFa, while their levels of RBC glutathione was higher in comparison to the placebo group. Also significant improvements in oxygenation was observed in the group taking the ginger. The authors in the study stated that a significant difference was exhibited in patients in the time spent in the intensive care and their dependence upon mechanical ventilation. The study also found that the patients taking ginger (Zingiber officinale) did not exhibit a reduction in organ failure, barotrauma or mortality compared to the placebo group was similar (*Vahdat Shariatpanahi et al., 2013*).

Chemical composition -
Gingerols, paradols, shogaols, wikstromol, and carinol (*Idris et al., 2019*).

Additional Herbs for Helping Fight COVID-19
Friedelanol which has been isolated from Euphorbia neriifolia and Blancoxanthone which has been isolated from the roots of Calophyllum blancoi has been shown to possess anti-HCoV-229E activity [27] [28].

Herbs used to fight the Influenza Virus
There currently exist metanalyses studies showing how effective herbs are at treating the flu (*Wagner L. et al., 2015; Ang et al., 2020b*).

The Lian Hua Qing Wen Capsule Formula
The formula known as Lian Hua Qing Wen Capsule was shown to inhibit the propagation of various influenza viruses. The herbal formula blocked the beginning stages of the influenza virus and also inhibited virus-induced gene expression of TNF-a, IP-10, IL-6, IL-8 and MCP-1 [29].

Herbs used to combat the 2003 SARS Pandemic
The Dayuan Decoction (DYD)
From the months of January to April 2003, 112 SARS cases were treated with the Dayuan Decoction. 93.7% of the patients experienced symptoms of a reduction in their illness and recovery [29a].

The Dayuan decoction is currently being used as a treatment for COVID-19 in China. The formula is composed of Ephedra (sinica Stapf herb), Areca catechu L, Magnolia officinalis Rehder and E.H.Wilson herbs, Atractylodes macrocephala (Koidz herb), Citrus reticulata Blanco, Amomum tsao-ko Crevost et Lemaire, Zingiber officinale Rosc (common ginger), Citrus aurantium L, Pogostemon cablin (Blanco) Benth, Hansenia weberbaueriana (Fedde ex H.Wolff) Pimenov and Kljuykov herbs. The mass ratios used are 10: 10: 15: 10: 6: 6: 10: 10:10 [29b].

A scientific team reviewed three studies that used TCM for the prevention of SARS as well as 4 studies for the prevention of H1N1 influenza. The study found that none of the participants who took TCM contracted SARS in three of the studies and that the infection rate of H1N1 in the group who used TCM was significantly lower than the non-TCM group. The main principles of the herbs were to resolve dampness, to tonify qi to protect from external pathogens, discharge heat and to disperse wind. The herbs used the most were Radix glycyrrhizae (Gancao), Radix saposhnikoviae (Fangfeng), Radix astragali (Huangqi), Rhizoma Atractylodis Macrocephalae (Baizhu), Lonicerae Japonicae Flos (Jinyinhua) and Fructus forsythia (Lianqiao) [29c].

In a high-profile study published in the Lancet, researchers reported that glycyrrhizin, which is an active constituent in the herb liquorice root, was the most frequently used Chinese herb used to inhibit replication of the SARS virus. In another study researchers discovered that the Chinese herbal compound baicalin exhibited anti-SARS activity [30] [31].

The Chinese Rhubarb extract
The following herbal extracts have been shown to inhibit the enzymatic activity of SARS 3CLpro:

Chinese Rhubarb extracts [32] (IC50: 13.76 ± 0.03 µg/mL)

A water extract of Houttuynia cordata [33] [34].

A Flavonoid extracted from litchi seeds [35]

Beta-sitosterol (IC50: 1210µM) extracted from the root extract of Isatis indigotica [36].

Indigo Dye
Semisynthetic diversely substituted analogues of isatin, which is a tiny natural molecule derived from purple dye indigo, was found to be very active towards 3CLpro. It's IC50 ranged from the lower micromolar range (0.95 µM) up to 23.5 µM [37] [38].

Also extracts of Sinomenium acutum (IC50:198.6 μg/mL), Coriolus versicolor (IC50:108.4 μg/mL), Kang Du Bu Fei Tang (IC50:471.3 μg/mL) and Ganoderma lucidum (IC50:41.9 μg/mL) have been shown to inhibit SARS-CoV RdRp in a dose- dependent manner [39].

Herbs shown to inhibit SARS 3CLpro activity [40] [41] [42]
The naturally occurring compounds of -

quercetin (IC50: 73μM)
epigallocatechin gallate (IC50: 73μM)
gallocatechin gallate (IC50: 47 μM)
sinigrin (IC50: 217μM)
indigo (IC50: 752μM)
aloe-emodin (IC50: 366 μM)
hesperetin (IC50:8.3 μM)

herbacetin
rhoifolin
pectolinarin

Indigo in Detail
Methanol extracts of indiindium and indigo were found to inhibit the activity of the Japanese encephalitis virus (JEV). It was also found to be less cytotoxic than other components. Indiindium showed rather strong protective effects on mice that were indirectly infected with JEV (*Chang et al., 2012*). The researchers discovered that indiindium did not directly inhibit the virus per say, but actually but inhibited the expression of activated chemokines in human bronchial epithelial cells that were infected with influenza virus. Activated chemokines exist as normal T cells and a secretory factor RANTES (*Mak et al., 2004*).

Substances that Inhibit SARS-CoV replication [43]

A research study performed a large scale meta-screening of over 10,000 substances, looking for the ones that exhibited anti-SARS-CoV activity. The study discovered the following substances exhibited the best effects -

Aescin, isolated from the horse chestnut tree.

Ginsenoside-Rb1, isolated from ginseng.

Reserpine contained in the genus Rauwolfia.

Extracts of eucalyptus and Lonicera japonica.

Escin

Escin exhibits anti-inflammatory, antiedematous and antioxidant properties and is widely used for treating traumatic edema and hemorrhoids; without adverse side effects. A study stated that Escin's inflammatory properties may play potential roles in treating COVID-19 patients and that the antiviral drug, such as remdesivir, or in combination with escin may exhibit therapeutic effects in severe COVID-19 patients [43a].

Other Potential anti-SARS-CoV Herbs

Emodin from Rheum and Polygonum [44]

Baicalin from Scutellaria baicalensis [45] [46]

Baicalin in detail

Baicalin is extracted from the Scutellaria genus and

Erigerontis herba (Dengzhanxixin or Dengzhanhua in Chinese) and exhibits anti- apoptotic activity. It is used to treat pulmonary atrial hypertension. Chen et al. (*2004*) discovered that Baicalin exhibits anti-SARS-CoV activity via an inhibitory effect. S. baicalensis extracts exhibit broad spectrum anti-viral activities against H1N123, HIV24, ZIKA22, and DENV25. An in-depth analysis showed that S. baicalensis exhibited stronger antiviral effects and better clinical efficacy than ribavirin for treating of hand, foot, and mouth disease [46a]. Hence, certain S. baicalensis compounds have been approved for use as antiviral drugs. These include the Huangqin tablet (to treat upper respiratory infection and the Baicalein capsule (to treat hepatitis).

A research study looked at S. baicalensis extract as well as the four active baicalein compounds present (S. baicalensis: baicalin, wogonin, baicalein and wogonoside) in vitro, looking at their effectiveness against SARS-CoV 3CLpro in vitro. The study found that Baicalein showed the most potent anti-SARS-CoV-2 3Clpro [46b].

Nicotianamine from soybeans [47]

Scutellarin [48]

Tetra-O-galloyl-β-D-glucose (TGG) from Galla chinensis and luteolin from Veronicalina riifolia [49]

Quercetin Exhibits potent Anti-Sars Activity
The substance TSL-1 and Quercetin extracted from Toona sinensis Roem showed potent anti-SARS-CoV effects [50].
When quercetin and TSL-1 was extracted from Toona sinensis Roem it exhibited the ability to inhibit SARS coronavirus replication via entry, adsorption and penetration [50a].

Further Reading
Traditional Chinese Medicine in the Treatment of Patients Infected with 2019-New Coronavirus (SARS-CoV-2): A Review and Perspective

Additional Herbs and Substances to reduce COVID-19 Infection

Oleandrin
Researchers discovered that when cells were treated in test tubes with oleandrin, either before or after exposure to SARS-CoV-2, which is the virus that causes COVID-19, that it reduced the production of the virus 78-fold to 800-fold (*Plante, bioRxiv 2020*).

Please Note - Ingestion of purified oleander can be highly toxic. Some people have died after ingesting oleander, either accidentally or intentionally. The toxicity is attributed to the cardiac glycosides in oleander (*Azzalini, J Forensic Leg Med 2019*).

Minerals and Vitamins for COVID-19 defense

Vitamin K (*found in abundance in raw Kale and Natto*)
Lower Vitamin K levels in the body have been associated with an increased risk of contracting COVID-19 as well as experiencing unfavorable outcomes from the disease.

Vitamin C
An above average intake of Vitamin C may help people who are critically ill with COVID-19. A review of several studies found a daily dose of 1,000 to 6,000 mg of vitamin C taken

either by mouth or intravenously shortened the time on ventilation by about 25% (*Hemila J Intens Care 2020*).

Selenium

A study conducted in Germany (*Selenium Deficiency Is Associated with Mortality Risk from COVID-19. Arash Moghaddam et al. July 2020*) found that selenium deficiency was a common trait in people that were diagnosed with COVID-19, and that it is more common among those who die from COVID-19.

Researchers discovered to their surprise that when selenium was given to selenium-deficient patients that it increased enhanced their immune system to viral infections. The study also found that it decreased the virulence of several viruses and in certain cases to the point of complete prevention of their disease (*Guillin O, Vindry C, Ohlmann T, Chavatte L. Selenium, selenoproteins and viral infection. Nutrients 2019;11:E2101. doi:10.3390/nu11092101*).

Selenium is anti-inflammatory and supports the body's antioxidant system. Higher doses have been shown to enhance the body's resistance against foreign viruses and bad bacteria (*Rayman, 2012*). Other studies have found it enhances the body's immune system (*Broome et al., 2004*) including that of poliovirus (*Ivory et al., 2017*).

Zinc

A research study by Acevedo-Murillo et al. (*2019*), involving 103 children that had pneumonia symptoms showed improvement in rate of respiration, oxygen saturation and the duration of illness when taking zinc, compared to the control group.

People particularly at risk for low zinc in their diets include vegetarians or people taking specific prescription medications (*such as stomach acid medications or ACE inhibitors*).

Research has also shown that taking a zinc supplement at 20 mg per day may improve the chance of avoiding respiratory tract infections. This was shown in a study of elderly people in French nursing facilities. The participants were also found to be deficient in selenium and were given 100 mcg per day of selenium orally during the study.

In a research study, zinc inhibited the replication of coronaviruses in cells [52].

In another case, a physician reported that four people with COVID-19 reported significant improvements in their health in only 24 hours after taking zinc lozenges. This however was not a controlled clinical study [53].

Cautions about using Zinc
Zinc can impair the absorption of some prescription antibiotics. The daily doses of zinc in zinc lozenges usually exceed the tolerable upper limits for zinc. Hence, they should not be taken longer than about a week.

Further Reading
Treatment of SARS-CoV-2 with high dose oral zinc salts: A report on four patients Eric Finzi.

Elderberry Extract
While Elderberry extract is one of nature's most powerful flu fighters, it is a double edged sword and should be used with caution. Elderberry extract may cause a cytokine storm reaction in people diagnosed with COVID-19. However a study showed that it has powerful anti-viral properties [54].

The latest studies on Chloroquine and Hydroxychloroquine for Defeating COVID-19

Chloroquine

Chloroquine exists as an ant malarial drug, developed in 1934. Anti-malarials are some of the most potent weapons one can use to fight COVID-19. Cinchona trees (Chincona L., Raiatea) grow in the remote Andean mountain forests. These trees contain bioactive compounds which can heal fevers and chills (*C. Maldonado et al. 2017*).

Quinine Alkaloids

The bark of Cinchona produces quinine alkaloids which have been shown to be very effective in treating malaria for more than several centuries. Quinine's behavior is similar to chloroquine, the synthetic antimalaria substance used for treating malaria (chloroquine analogue). To date, Quinine sulphate is one of the most sought after substances for treating COVID-19 [55].

Quinine Reactions

A research review study by Liles et al. discovered that a couple of general adverse reactions have been demonstrated by quinine; such as toxic and immune-mediated reactions [56]. Hence continued routine consumption of Cinchona should be used with extreme caution for healthy people seeking to prevent becoming infected with COVID-19 because of the possibility that it may lead to certain harmful events.

Hydroxychloroquine

Hydroxychloroquine is used to treat autoimmune diseases and was developed in 1946. It exists as an analogue of chloroquine. Both hydroxychloroquine and chloroquine exhibit antiviral activity in certain in vitro systems (*Chloroquine or Hydroxychloroquine With or Without Azithromycin. www.nih.gov*). Both Hydroxychloroquine and Chloroquine when used with or without azithromycin, have been tested in multiple clinical trials for treating COVID-19. The most recent clinical stated that hydroxychloroquine was ineffective (*Geleris et al., 2020*).

Additionally, in a large controlled trial of patients hospitalized with COVID-19 in the United Kingdom, hydroxychloroquine was found to not decrease the 28-day mortality, compared to standard care (*Chloroquine or Hydroxychloroquine With or Without Azithromycin. www.nih.gov*).

Another controlled trial conducted in Brazil discovered that neither hydroxychloroquine alone nor hydroxychloroquine with azithromycin improved the clinical outcomes of hospitalized patients diagnosed with mild to moderate COVID-19 (*Chloroquine or Hydroxychloroquine With or Without Azithromycin. www.nih.gov*).

In another a large observational study of patients hospitalized with COVID-19, hydroxychloroquine was not associated with reduced risks of death or the need for ventilation (*Chloroquine or Hydroxychloroquine With or Without Azithromycin. www.nih.gov*).

How effective is Remdesevir?

In a placebo controlled trial, remdesevir exhibited a significant reduction in the mortality of COVID-19 patients (1063 patients) (*Beigel et al., 2020*). In a later Phase 3 clinical trial (SIMPLE) the study showed a 62% reduction in mortality.

Chlorine Dioxide

Although there are no confirmed studies as of yet, chlorine dioxide that has been properly diluted with water by adding just a few drops to a cup of distilled water has yielded many online testimonials. This homemade version is called Miracle Mineral Solution or MMS for short. Chlorine Dioxide is usually made by mixing Lemon Juice (citric acid) with a small amount of Sodium Chlorite and then adding a few drops of this solution to a cup of distilled water.

MMS is banned for commercial sale in the USA Anyone that is caught making the Chlorine Dioxide version known as Miracle Mineral Solution (MMS) and then selling it in the United States has been questioned by authorities and in some cases sent to court. It is however legal to sell Miracle Mineral Solution in New Zealand; one of the countries with the lowest rates of COVID-19 to date.

Numbered References. Chapter 9

(27) Chang FR, Yen CT, Ei-Shazly M, Lin WH, Yen MH, Lin KH. et al. Anti-Human Coronavirus (anti-HCoV) Triterpenoids from the Leaves of Euphorbia Neriifolia. Nat Prod Commun. 2012;7:1934578X1200701103.

(28) Shen YC, Wang LT, Khalil AT, Chiang LC, Cheng PW. Bioactive Pyranoxanthones from the Roots of Calophyllum blancoi. Chem Pharm Bull. 2005;53:244-7.

(29) Ding Y, Zeng L, Li R, Chen Q, Zhou B, Chen Q. et al. The Chinese prescription lianhuaqingwen capsule exerts anti-influenza activity through the inhibition of viral propagation and impacts immune function. BMC Complement Altern Med. 2017;17:130.

(29a) X.R. Zhang, T.N. Li, Y.Y. Ren, Y.J. Zeng, H.Y. Lv, J. Wang, Q.W. Huang, The important role of volatile components from a traditional chinese medicine dayuan-yin against the COVID-19 pandemic, Front. Pharmacol. 11 (2020), 583651.

(29b) Research progress of traditional Chinese medicine against COVID-19. Wei Ren et al. February 2021.

(29c) Can Chinese Medicine Be Used for Prevention of Corona Virus Disease 2019 (COVID-19)? A Review of Historical Classics, Research Evidence and Current Prevention Programs. Hui Luo et al. Feb 2020.

(30) Cinatl J, Morgenstern B, Bauer G, Chandra P, Rabenau H, Doerr HW. Glycyrrhizin, an active component of liquorice roots, and replication of SARS-associated coronavirus. The Lancet. 2003;361:2045-6.

(31) Chen F, Chan KH, Jiang Y, Kao RY, Lu HT, Fan KW. et al. In vitro susceptibility of 10 clinical isolates of SARS coronavirus to selected antiviral compounds. J Clin Virol. 2004;31:69-75.

(32) Luo W, Su X, Gong S, Qin Y, Liu W, Li J, Anti-SARS coronavirus 3C-like protease effects of Rheum palmatum L. extracts. BioScience Trends. 2009.

(33) Fung KP, Leung PC, Tsui KW, Wan CC, Wong KB, Waye MY. et al. Immunomodulatory activities of the herbal formula Kwan Du Bu Fei Dang in healthy subjects: a randomised, double-blind, placebo-controlled study. Hong Kong Med J. 2011;17(Suppl 2):41-3.

(34) Lau KM, Lee KM, Koon CM, Cheung CS, Lau CP, Ho HM. et al. Immunomodulatory and anti-SARS activities of Houttuynia cordata. J Ethnopharmacol. 2008;118:79-85.

(35) Gong SJ, Su XJ, Yu HP, Li J, Qin YJ, Xu Q. et al. A study on anti-SARS-CoV 3CL protein of flavonoids from litchi chinensis sonn core. Chinese Pharmacological Bulletin. 2008;24:699-700.

(36) Lin CW, Tsai FJ, Tsai CH, Lai CC, Wan L, Ho TY. et al. Anti-SARS coronavirus 3C-like protease effects of Isatis indigotica root and plant-derived phenolic compounds. Antiviral Res. 2005;68:36-42.

(37) Chen, L.-R.; Wang, Y.-C.; Lin, Y.W.; Chou, S.-Y.; Chen, S.-F.; Liu, L.T.; Wu, Y.-T.; Kuo, C.-J.; Chen, T.S.-S.; Juang, S.-H. Synthesis and evaluation of isatin derivatives as effective SARS coronavirus 3CL protease inhibitors. Bioorg. Med. Chem. Lett. 2005, 15, 3058-3062.

(38) Liu, W.; Zhu, H.-M.; Niu, G.-J.; Shi, E.-Z.; Chen, J.; Sun, B.; Chen, W.; Zhou, H.; Yang, C. Synthesis, modification and docking studies of 5-sulfonyl isatin derivatives as SARS-CoV 3C-like protease inhibitors. Bioorg. Med. Chem. 2014, 22, 292-302.

(39) Fung KP, Leung PC, Tsui KW, Wan CC, Wong KB, Waye MY. et al. Immunomodulatory activities of the herbal formula Kwan Du Bu Fei Dang in healthy subjects: a randomised, double-blind, placebo-controlled study. Hong Kong Med J. 2011;17(Suppl 2):41-3.

(40) Nguyen TTH, Woo HJ, Kang HK, Nguyen VD, Kim YM, Kim DW. et al. Flavonoid-mediated inhibition of SARS coronavirus 3C-like protease expressed in Pichia pastoris. Biotechnol Lett. 2012;34:831-8.

(41) Jo S, Kim S, Shin DH, Kim M-S. Inhibition of SARS-CoV 3CL protease by flavonoids. J Enzyme Inhib Med Chem. 2020;35:145-51.

(42) Jo S, Kim H, Kim S, Shin DH, Kim MS. Characteristics of flavonoids as potent MERS-CoV 3C-like protease inhibitors. Chem Biol Drug Des. 2019.

(43) Wu CY, Jan JT, Ma SH, Kuo CJ, Juan HF, Cheng YSE. et al. Small molecules targeting severe acute respiratory syndrome human coronavirus. Proc Natl Acad Sci U S A. 2004;101:10012-7.

(43a) Severe Acute Lung Injury Related to COVID-19 Infection: A Review and the Possible Role for Escin. Luca Gallelli,. et al. May 2020.

(44) Ho T, Wu S, Chen J, Li C, Hsiang C. Emodin blocks the SARS coronavirus spike protein and angiotensin-converting enzyme 2 interaction. Antiviral Res. 2007;74:92-101.

(45) Chen Z, Nakamura T. Statistical evidence for the usefulness of Chinese medicine in the treatment of SARS. Phytotherapy research: PTR. 2004;18:592-4.

(46) Deng YF, Aluko RE, Jin Q, Zhang Y, Yuan LJ. Inhibitory activities of baicalin against renin and angiotensin-converting enzyme. Pharm Biol. 2012;50:401-6.

(46a) Lin H, Zhou J, Lin K, et al. Efficacy of Scutellaria baicalensis for the treatment of hand, foot, and mouth disease associated with encephalitis in patients infected with EV71: a multicenter, retrospective analysis. Biomed Res Int 2016;2016: 5697571).

(46b) Scutellaria baicalensis extract and baicalein inhibit replication of SARS-CoV-2 and its 3C-like protease in vitro. Hongbo Liua et al. Journal Of Enzyme Inhibition And Medicinal Chemistry 2021, VOL. 36, NO. 1, 497–503.

(47) Takahashi S, Yoshiya T, Yoshizawa-Kumagaye K, Sugiyama T. Nicotianamine is a novel angiotensin-converting enzyme 2 inhibitor in soybean. Biomed Res. 2015;36:219-24.

(48) Wang W, Ma X, Han J, Zhou M, Ren H, Pan Q. et al. Neuroprotective Effect of Scutellarin on Ischemic Cerebral Injury by Down-Regulating the Expression of Angiotensin-Converting Enzyme and AT1 Receptor. PLoS One. 2016;11:e0146197.

(49) Yi L, Li Z, Yuan K, Qu X, Chen J, Wang G. et al. Small molecules blocking the entry of severe acute respiratory syndrome coronavirus into host cells. J Virol. 2004;78:11334-9.

(50) Chen CJ, Michaelis M, Hsu HK, Tsai CC, Yang KD, Wu YC. et al. Toona sinensis Roem tender leaf extract inhibits SARS coronavirus replication. J Ethnopharmacol. 2008;120:108-11.

(50a) Chen CJ, Michaelis M, Hsu HK, Tsai CC, Yang KD, Wu YC, et al. Toona sinensis Roem tender leaf extract inhibits SARS coronavirus replication. J Ethnopharmacol. 2008; 120: 108-11.

(51) A cohort study to evaluate the effect of combination Vitamin D, Magnesium and Vitamin B12 (DMB) on progression to severe outcome in older COVID-19 patients. JUne 2020.

(52) Zn2+ Inhibits Coronavirus and Arterivirus RNA Polymerase Activity In Vitro and Zinc Ionophores Block the Replication of These Viruses in Cell Culture. Aartjan J. et al.

(53) Treatment of SARS-CoV-2 with high dose oral zinc salts: A report on four patients Author links open overlay panel. EricFinzi.

(54) The effect of Sambucol, a black elderberry-based, natural product, on the production of human cytokines: I. Inflammatory cytokines. V Barak et al. June 2001.

(55) E. Abolghasemi, S. H. Moosa-Kazemi, M. Davoudi, A. Reisi, and M. T. Satvat, "Comparative study of chloroquine and quinine on malaria rodents and their effects on the mouse testis," Asian Pacific Journal of Tropical Biomedicine, vol. 2, no. 4, pp. 311–314, 2012.

(56) N. W.Liles,E.E. Page,A.L. Liles,S.K. Vesely, G. E.Raskob, and J. N. George, "Diversity and severity of adverse reactions to quinine: a systematic review," American Journal of Hematology, vol. 91, no. 5, pp. 461–466, 2016.

Chapter 10. Anti-HCoV agents active against anti-SARS-CoV activity and the common cold.

These agents are known in the scientific literature as HCoVs, 229E, NL63, OC43 and HKU1. The following is a list of the best herbs shown to inhibit these agents.

In a recent screening for broad spectrum anti-HCoV agents against NL63, OC43 and MERS, the alkaloids lycorine and emetine showed it inhibited viral replication of all strains with EC50 below 5 μM [1].

Chamaecyparis obtusa (Cupressaceae)
The abietane diterpene ferruginol isolated from Chamaecyparis obtusa (Cupressaceae) has exhibited an EC50 of 1.39 μM. Whereas the labdane diterpene pinusolidic acid was shown to inhibit SARS-CoV infection at an EC50 of 4.71 μM and an excellent SI [2] [3].

Strobilanthes cusia (Acanthaceae)
Indole alkaloids tryptanthrine and indigodole B isolated from Strobilanthes cusia (Acanthaceae) reduced NL63 in early and late stages of LLC-MJ2 cells infection. It also inhibited the enzymes responsible for viral replication (PLP2, RNTylophora indica (Apocynaceae). Tylophorine and tylophorine N-oxide extracted from Tylophora indica (Apocynaceae) has shown notable anti-SARS-CoV activity due to the presence of phenanthraindolizidine alkaloids tylophorine [4].

Betulonic acid
Studies have found that the triterpene betulonic acid showed very good anti-SARS-CoV activity, with an EC50 of 0.63 µM [5] [6] [7] [8] [9].

Euphorbia neriifolia
Pentacyclic triterpenes isolated from Euphorbia neriifolia (Euphorbiaceae) exhibited anti-HCov potential [10].

Xanthones isolated from Calophyllum blancoi (Guttiferae) [11].

Favagline silvestrol isolated from plants of the genus Aglaia (Meliaceae) [12].

Silvestrol
Silvestrol shows an EC50 in the nanomolar range. It shows no significant cytotoxic effect in the primary cells [13].

Tacrolimus
Tacrolimus is used as an immunosuppressant drug and comes from the soil bacterium Streptomyces tsukubaiensis [14].

The 3β-OH analogue of betulonic acid (betulinic acid), has exhibited weak antiviral activity (EC50 > 10 µM) and it strongly inhibited SARS-CoV 3CLpro (IC50 = 10 µM) [15].

Stephania tetrandra (Menispermaceae)
Cepharanthine, fangchinoline and tetrandrine is isolated from Stephania tetrandra (Menispermaceae). It has been shown to inhibit the OC-43 induced cell death of lung cells, during early infection as well as suppress viral replication [16] [17].

An extract of Pelargoniumsidoides (Geraniaceae) exhibited weak activity against 229E (EC50 = 44.50 µg/mL) and was approved in Germany for treating respiratory infections at 44.50 µg/Ml [18].

The Natural Products Guestrin, 3-theaflavin-3-gallate and Amentoflavone

Tripterygium regeli (Celastraceae)
Among numerous NPs tested, the pentacyclic triterpene iguestrin, extracted from the root of Tripterygium regeli (Celastraceae) showed the best activity with an IC50 of 2.6 µM. This was followed by pristimerin (5.5 µM) [19].

Amentoflavone at (8.3 µM) [20].

3-theaflavin-3-gallate at (9.8 µM) [21].

Salvia miltiorrhiza (Lamiaceae)
The tanshinone derivatives extracted from Salvia miltiorrhiza (Lamiaceae) has been shown to exhibit excellent inhibitory activity against PLpro (papain-like protease). Cryptotanshinone exhibited an IC50 of 0.8 µM [22].

Angelica keiskei (Apiaceae)
A chalcone derivative isolated from the leaves extract of Angelica keiskei (Apiaceae) in extract form showed an IC50 of 1.2 µM [23].

Myricetin and Scutellarein
Just one study exists investigating the inhibition of SARS-CoV helicase from NPs. The flavonoids myricetin and scutellarein inhibited nsp13 with IC50 0.86 and 2.71 µM, respectively [24].

Parthenolide
This natural product was shown to inhibit all three Janus kinases (JAK1, JAK2 andTYK2) inhibiting overall STAT3 signaling [25].

Further Reading
Janus kinase inhibitors for the treatment of rheumatoid arthritis demonstrate similar profiles of in vitro cytokine receptor inhibition. Dowty, M.E.; Lin, T.H.; Jesson, M.I.; Hegen, M.; Martin, D.A.; Katkade, V.; Menon, S.; Telliez, J. Pharmacol. Res. Perspect. 2019, 7, e00537.

Natural and Nature-Derived Products Targeting Human Coronaviruses. Konstantina Vougogiannopoulou et al. Jan 2021. Department of Pharmacognosy and Natural Products Chemistry, Faculty of Pharmacy, National and Kapodistrian University of Athens, Panepistimiopolis Zografou, 15771 Athens, Greece.

Other substances obtained from plants (*and some manufactured*) that exhibit anti-SARS-CoV activity [26] with EC50 close to or below the 10μM range include -

reserpine
β-yohimbine
gallicacid
honokiol
forskolin
magnolol

Numbered References. Chapter 10

(1) Shen, L.; Niu, J.; Wang, C.; Huang, B.; Wang, W.; Zhu, N.; Deng, Y.; Wang, H.; Ye, F.; Cen, S.; et al. High-Throughput Screening and Identification of Potent Broad-Spectrum Inhibitors of Coronaviruses. J. Virol. 2019, 93.

(2) Khan, S.A.; Zia, K.; Ashraf, S.; Uddin, R.; Ul-Haq, Z. Identification of chymotrypsin-like protease inhibitors of SARS-CoV-2 via integrated computational approach. J. Biomol. Struct. Dyn. 2020, 1–10.

(3) Wen, C.-C.; Kuo, Y.-H.; Jan, J.-T.; Liang, P.-H.; Wang, S.-Y.; Liu, H.-G.; Lee, C.-K.; Chang, S.-T.; Kuo, C.-J.; Lee, S.-S.; et al. Specific Plant Terpenoids and Lignoids Possess Potent Antiviral Activities against Severe Acute Respiratory Syndrome Coronavirus. J. Med. Chem. 2007, 50, 4087–4095.

(4) Yang, C.-W.; Lee, Y.-Z.; Kang, I.-J.; Barnard, D.L.; Jan, J.-T.; Lin, D.; Huang, C.-W.; Yeh, T.-K.; Chao, Y.-S.; Lee, S.-J. Identification of phenanthroindolizines and phenanthroquinolizidines as novel potent anti-coronaviral agents for porcine enteropathogenic coronavirus transmissible gastroenteritis virus and human severe acute respiratory syndrome coronavirus. Antivir. Res. 2010, 88, 160–168.

(5) Wu, C.-Y.; Jan, J.-T.; Ma, S.-H.; Kuo, C.-J.; Juan, H.-F.; Cheng, Y.-S.E.; Hsu, H.-H.; Huang, H.-C.; Wu, D.; Brik, A.; et al. Small molecules targeting severe acute respiratory syndrome human coronavirus. Proc. Natl. Acad. Sci. USA 2004, 101, 10012–10017.

(6) Hoever, G.; Baltina, L.; Michaelis, M.; Kondratenko, R.; Tolstikov, G.A.; Doerr, H.W.; Cinatl, J. Antiviral Activity of Glycyrrhizic Acid Derivatives against SARS−Coronavirus. J. Med. Chem. 2005, 48, 1256–1259.

(7) Wen, C.-C.; Kuo, Y.-H.; Jan, J.-T.; Liang, P.-H.; Wang, S.-Y.; Liu, H.-G.; Lee, C.-K.; Chang, S.-T.; Kuo, C.-J.; Lee, S.-S.; et al. Specific

Plant Terpenoids and Lignoids Possess Potent Antiviral Activities against Severe Acute Respiratory Syndrome Coronavirus. J. Med. Chem. 2007, 50, 4087-4095.

(8) Kim, H.; Eo, E.-Y.; Park, H.; Kim, Y.-C.; Park, S.; Shin, H.; Kim, K. Medicinal herbal extracts of Sophorae radix, Acanthopanacis cortex, Sanguisorbae radix and Torilis fructus inhibit coronavirus replication in vitro. Antivir. Ther. 2010, 15, 697-709

(9) Cheng, P.-W.; Ng, L.-T.; Chiang, L.-C.; Lin, C.-C. Antiviral effects of saikosaponins on human coronavirus 229E in vitro. Clin. Exp. Pharmacol. Physiol. 2006, 33, 612-616).

(10) Chang, F.-R.; Yen, C.-T.; Ei-Shazly, M.; Lin, W.-H.; Yen, M.-H.; Lin, K.-H.; Wu, Y.-C. Anti-human coronavirus (anti-HCoV) triterpenoids from the leaves of Euphorbia neriifolia. Nat. Prod. Commun. 2012, 7, 1415-1417.

(11) Shen, Y.-C.; Wang, L.-T.; Khalil, A.T.; Chiang, L.C.; Cheng, P.-W. Bioactive pyranoxanthones from the roots of Calophyllum blancoi. Chem. Pharm. Bull. 2005, 53, 244-247.

(12) Müller, C.; Schulte, F.W.; Lange-Grünweller, K.; Obermann, W.; Madhugiri, R.; Pleschka, S.; Ziebuhr, J.; Hartmann, R.K.; Grünweller, A. Broad-spectrum antiviral activity of the eIF4A inhibitor silvestrol against corona- and picornaviruses. Antivir. Res. 2018, 150, 123-129.

(13) Müller, C.; Schulte, F.W.; Lange-Grünweller, K.; Obermann, W.; Madhugiri, R.; Pleschka, S.; Ziebuhr, J.; Hartmann, R.K.; Grünweller, A. Broad-spectrum antiviral activity of the eIF4A inhibitor silvestrol against corona- and picornaviruses. Antivir. Res. 2018, 150, 123-129.

(14) Hatanaka, H.; Iwami, M.; Kino, T.; Goto, T.; Okuhara, M. FR-900520 and FR-900523, novel immunosuppressants isolated from a Streptomyces. I. Taxonomy of the producing strain. J. Antibiot. (Tokyo) 1988, 41, 1586-1591.

(15) Wen, C.-C.; Kuo, Y.-H.; Jan, J.-T.; Liang, P.-H.; Wang, S.-Y.; Liu, H.-G.; Lee, C.-K.; Chang, S.-T.; Kuo, C.-J.; Lee, S.-S.; et al. Specific Plant Terpenoids and Lignoids Possess Potent Antiviral Activities against Severe Acute Respiratory Syndrome Coronavirus. J. Med. Chem. 2007, 50, 4087–4095.

(16) Kim, D.E.; Min, J.S.; Jang, M.S.; Lee, J.Y.; Shin, Y.S.; Park, C.M.; Song, J.H.; Kim, H.R.; Kim, S.; Jin, Y.-H.; et al. Natural bisbenzylisoquinoline alkaloids-tetrandrine, fangchinoline, and cepharanthine, inhibit human coronavirus oc43 infection of mrc-5 human lung cells. Biomolecules 2019, 9, 696.

(17) Shen, L.; Niu, J.; Wang, C.; Huang, B.; Wang, W.; Zhu, N.; Deng, Y.; Wang, H.; Ye, F.; Cen, S.; et al. High-Throughput Screening and Identification of Potent Broad-Spectrum Inhibitors of Coronaviruses. J. Virol. 2019, 93.

(18) Michaelis, M.; Doerr, H.W.; Cinatl, J. Investigation of the influence of EPs® 7630, a herbal drug preparation from Pelargonium sidoides, on replication of a broad panel of respiratory viruses. Phytomedicine 2011, 18, 384–386.

(19) Ryu, Y.B.; Park, S.-J.; Kim, Y.M.; Lee, J.-Y.; Seo, W.D.; Chang, J.S.; Park, K.H.; Rho, M.-C.; Lee, W.S. SARS-CoV 3CLpro inhibitory effects of quinone-methide triterpenes from Tripterygium regelii. Bioorg. Med. Chem. Lett. 2010, 20, 1873–1876.

(20) Ryu, Y.B.; Jeong, H.J.; Kim, J.H.; Kim, Y.M.; Park, J.-Y.; Kim, D.; Naguyen, T.T.H.; Park, S.-J.; Chang, J.S.; Park, K.H. Biflavonoids from Torreya nucifera displaying SARS-CoV 3CLpro inhibition. Bioorg. Med. Chem. 2010, 18, 7940–794

(21) Schmidtke, M.; Meier, C.; Schacke, M.; Helbig, B.; Makarov, V.; Rabenau, H.F.; Cinatl, J.; Wutzler, P. Antiviral activity of phenolic polymers and cycloSal-pronucleotides against a SARS-associated coronavirus. Chemother. J. 2005, 14, 16–21.

(22) Park, J.-Y.; Kim, J.H.; Kim, Y.M.; Jeong, H.J.; Kim, D.W.; Park, K.H.; Kwon, H.-J.; Park, S.-J.; Lee, W.S.; Ryu, Y.B. Tanshinones as selective and slow-binding inhibitors for SARS-CoV cysteine proteases. Bioorg. Med. Chem. 2012, 20, 5928–5935.

(23) Park, J.-Y.; Ko, J.-A.; Kim, D.W.; Kim, Y.M.; Kwon, H.-J.; Jeong, H.J.; Kim, C.Y.; Park, K.H.; Lee, W.S.; Ryu, Y.B. Chalcones isolated fromAngelica keiskeiinhibit cysteine proteases of SARS-CoV. J. Enzym. Inhib. Med. Chem. 2016, 31, 23–30.

(24) Yu, M.-S.; Lee, J.; Lee, J.M.; Kim, Y.; Chin, Y.-W.; Jee, J.-G.; Keum, Y.-S.; Jeong, Y.-J. Identification of myricetin and scutellarein as novel chemical inhibitors of the SARS coronavirus helicase, nsP13. Bioorg. Med. Chem. Lett. 2012, 22, 4049–4054.

(25) Liu, M.; Xiao, C.; Sun, M.; Tan, M.; Hu, L.; Yu, Q. Parthenolide Inhibits STAT3 Signaling by Covalently Targeting Janus Kinases. Molecules 2018, 23, 1478.

(26) Wen, C.-C.; Kuo, Y.-H.; Jan, J.-T.; Liang, P.-H.; Wang, S.-Y.; Liu, H.-G.; Lee, C.-K.; Chang, S.-T.; Kuo, C.-J.; Lee, S.-S.; et al. Specific Plant Terpenoids and Lignoids Possess Potent Antiviral Activities against Severe Acute Respiratory Syndrome Coronavirus. J. Med. Chem. 2007, 50, 4087–4095.

Chapter 11. Using Bald's Eyesalve to fight Antibiotic Resistant Bacteria.

Today with the rise of anti-resistant bacteria, medicine is always on the lookout for new types of disinfectant technologies. It is a real blessing to have the technology we do today to prove or disprove if something is valid or not. In the case of healing, we have thousands, if not millions of published reports on the effectiveness or un-effectiveness of various combinations of healing compounds. Many of these are made public at the National Institutes of Health website, which is where the study on Bald's Eyesalve, which we are about to discuss is available for viewing.

What if we could look at healing formulas used in Europe during the Middle Ages. The middle ages in Europe began in the 5th century and lasted until approximately the 15th century. The middle ages is marked by the fall of the Western Roman Empire, which then merged into the Renaissance and Age of Discovery. It was a time where new discoveries were being made, much like today. During the middle ages infections were one of the most feared superbugs. Most notably the Black Plague which lasted from 1346-1353 killed millions of people. It was during this time a formula surfaced that involved a simple mixture of garlic, onion and wine. The name of the formula is known as Bald's Eyesalve. The formula was discovered in the British Library in a 10th century text known as Bald's Leechbook, which is widely considered to be one of the earliest known medical textbooks, making it a formula over 1,000 years old. The formula was also considered to be the "*best of leechdoms*"   healing   remedies.

Reference
A 1,000-Year-Old Antimicrobial Remedy with Antistaphylococcal Activity. Published Jul/Aug 2015. Freya Harrison et al.

The formula was made to heal eye infections, which are similar in composition to germs/bugs that cause staph infections. Scientists wanted to test the formula to see if it would kill the Methicillin-resistant Staphylococcus aureus (MRSA) infection. This infection is caused by staph bacteria that has become resistant to antibiotics that are used to treat staph infections, making it a kind of modern-day superbug.

Scientists from the microbiology department of the University of Nottingham recreated the remedy and its preparation instructions, including the proper ratios of ingredients (such as using a brass vessel to brew it in) as closely as possible then tested the 1,000 year old formula on large cultures of MRSA.

Part of the instructions called for the formula to stand for nine days, at which time it was to be strained through a cloth (light fermentation) and to use wine from a vineyard known to have existed in the ninth century.

After microbiologists tested the formula on MRSA, methicillin-resistant Staphylococcus aureus (which is a staph bacterium that is ineffective to commonly used antibiotic treatments), they were astonished by the lab results.

The microbiologists reached the conclusion that Bald's Eyesalve was as effective as a prescription based antibiotic such as flucloxacillin or dicloxacillin, which are pharmaceutical based remedies used for treating serious MSSA infections. The microbiologists also asked a U.S. team to run the same tests on live mice. The results were the same. The microbiologists also found that Bald's Eyesalve keeps for a long period of time when stored in a refrigerator.

The conclusion of this scientific study? Bald's Eyesalve kills up to 90% of MRSA bacteria and that it is as effective as a prescription based antibiotic such as flucloxacillin or dicloxacillin.

In conclusion we can learn a lot from the masters of medicine during the middle ages (also known as the "dark ages". They lived in a period where they needed remedies that were effective to treat all sorts of plagues and infections. Bald's Eyesalve is just one example of this.

Chapter 12. Facts about Chlorine Dioxide.

In articles published in the New York Times on August 22, 2020 and in Reuters on October 30, 2020 the reporters stated that the Bolivian Congress (www.diputados.bo) authorized the use for the commercialization, supply and administration of diluted Chlorine Dioxide for use as a treatment for patients diagnosed with Coronavirus (COVID-19). When I fact checked this information for myself by going to the Bolivian Congress (www.diputados.bo) website, I discovered that the Bolivian Congress had authorized the use of Chlorine Dioxide on August 5th, 2020. The Bill stated that public and private laboratories accredited by the appropriate governing body can prepare Chlorine Dioxide Solution and distribute it with product leaflets that state the proper dosage and precautions when consuming and using the compound. Article 9 of the Bill stated that medical professionals can administer Chlorine Dioxide Solution with informed consent of the patient or a relative. The president of the Education and Health Commission, Deputy Franklin Flores, stated that this Bill will help give the population an alternative to face the Coronavirus pandemic.

The City of Sacramento California approves the use of Chlorine Dioxide for Killing COVID-19 Germs
During 2020, the city of Sacramento began using diluted Chlorine Dioxide to kill COVID-19 in many of its mass transit systems. Chlorine dioxide tablets are added to water in order to create a 400 parts per million diluted solution. Next an air fogger is used to spray public transportation vehicles. The entire process takes approximately seven minutes to fog a bus and up to 10 minutes completely to

disinfect passenger train carriages. After the spray particles have landed on seats and other regions, it takes approximately 30 minutes for the solution to completely dry, during which time the chlorine dioxide has killed germs.

Chlorine Dioxide is Cost Effective over the Long Term During the COVID-19 pandemic the price of some disinfectants has risen due to demand, as well as inflation. One of these is bleach. Chlorine Dioxide can be made affordably in large batches and it keeps for a long period of time, making it a very economical method of destroying bad viruses.

A Chlorine Dioxide Gargle that may Kill the COVID-19 Virus
Japanese researchers discovered that regular gargling with drinking water reduced incidences of upper respiratory tract infections to significant extent. The effect was because the drinking water in that Japanese district used contained 0.5 mg/L of chlorine, which was used to disinfect the drinking water [1].

Chlorine Dioxide is Scientifically Proven to Kill Viruses
In a research study published in 2020 titled: *Can chlorine dioxide prevent the spreading of coronavirus or other viral infections? Medical hypotheses*, that was conducted by K. KALY-KULLAI and colleagues at the Institute of Translational Medicine and International Nephrology Research and Training Center in Budapest, Hungary, the researchers state that an aqueous solution of Chlorine Dioxide kills and inactivates all types of viruses recommending it as a disinfectant in water, with a CT value of 8.4 mg 3 min/L, which is necessary to achieve a four-orders-of-magnitude ("4 log" or "99.99%") inactivation of bad bacterial viruses in an aqueous medium at a temperature of 25 8C [1a].

The study goes on to state that chlorine dioxide gas (that is moisturized) can be used against viruses in their wet and dry states; also killing viruses that are carried by water droplets in the air owing to the high solubility of ClO2 in water. The paper warns against using a dry ClO2 gas because the aqueous droplets could evaporate, slowing down the beneficial reactions necessary for killing bad bacteria. The paper also states that high concentrations of Chlorine Dioxide provide rapid disinfection of rooms when people are not present; making it useful for intensive care units, regions in quarantine or on public transport vessels. The application of chlorine dioxide when used as a gas spray is dangerous because it tends to gather in highly concentrated forms in enclosed spaces. The study concludes by stating Chlorine Dioxide can be useful as a preventive tool against influenza frequented by human activity. Attempts have been made to decrease the incidence of influenza among schoolchildren by applying low concentrations of chlorine dioxide gas in vacant classrooms [1a].

Dental Uses of Chlorine Dioxide in Preventing the Spread of Coronavirus (COVID-19)
Chlorine Dioxide has also been found to be of extreme benefit in preventing the spread of Coronavirus (COVID-19) when used in dental applications [2] [3].

The main component of Chlorine Dioxide is Sodium Chlorite. According to Wikipedia Sodium Chlorite is used for disinfection in municipal water treatment plants and when combined with zinc chloride, is used in toothpaste and mouthwashes. There is even a nasal spray that uses Sodium Chlorite and in the mid-2020's the city of Sacramento California began using chlorine dioxide to kill coronavirus on surfaces. And as of September 2020, the

Chinese have begun tests of a COVID-19 nasal spray vaccine (*China Starts Testing Covid-19 Nasal Spray Vaccine. Bloomberg News. September 10, 2020*).

Chlorine Dioxide (properly diluted in water) kills planktonic bacteria
A 1982 research study stated that solutions of Chlorine Dioxide (properly diluted in water) kills planktonic bacteria in a fraction of a second, making it safe to consume in very small amounts [3a]. Drinking 1 L of 24 mg/L ClO2 solution in two portions in one day has exhibited no observable negative outcomes effects in humans.

Further Reading
Can chlorine dioxide prevent the spreading of coronavirus or other viral infections? Кály-Kullai, K & Wittmann, Maria & Noszticzius, Z & Rosivall, Laszlo. (2020).

Raymond Tellier, a microbiologist at McGill University Health Center states that Coronavirus may be spreading through tiny aerosol particles which penetrate deep into the lungs, triggering severe infections. In summary, Chlorine Dioxide may be of great value to kill airborne particles of COVID-19 as long as the Chlorine Dioxide is properly diluted in distilled water and allowed to be exposed to open air in a very well ventilated area. This also means it may work well as a spray sanitizer. However in areas that do not have good ventilation, excessive inhalation of Chlorine Dioxide gas in an enclosed space has resulted in at least 1 documented case of human death [4].

Another research study found that those exposed to chlorine dioxide in the workplace exhibited susceptibility to chronic bronchitis and wheezing attacks but not for asthma [5].

Further Reading
Study on encapsulation of chlorine dioxide in gelatin microsphere for reducing release rate. Ying Ci et al.

Chlorine Dioxide Is a Size-Selective Antimicrobial Agent. Zoltán Nosziczius et al. Chlorine Dioxide Gas and its Protective Effect against Influenza

A 2017 research study conducted by Norio Ogata of the Taiko Pharmaceutical Corporation in Japan concluded that chlorine dioxide (ClO2) gas of extremely low concentrations exhibited zero toxic effects in experiments conducted on animals and shows strong anti-microbial activity against infectious microbes, such as bacteria and viruses [6].

Further Reading
Chlorine Dioxide (CLO2) As a Non-Toxic Antimicrobial Agent for Virus, Bacteria and Yeast.

Another research study involving mice concluded that chlorine dioxide gas exhibited protective effects against the influenza A Virus [7].

Further Reading
Antiviral Effect of Chlorine Dioxide against Influenza Virus and Its Application for Infection Control. Takanori Miura and Takashi Shibata. 2010.

Inactivation of a Human Norovirus Surrogate by Chlorine Dioxide Gas and Prediction of Human Norovirus Contamination by a Fecal Indicator System (Thesis)

Inactivation of human and simian rotaviruses by chlorine dioxide. Appl Environ Microbiol 56:1363-1366. Chen Y. S., Vaughn J. M. 1990.

Effect of chlorine dioxide gas on fungi and mycotoxins associated with sick building syndrome. Appl Environ Microbiol 71:5399-5403. Wilson S. C., Wu C., Andriychuk L. A., Martin J. M., Brasel T. L., Jumper C. A., Straus D. C. 2005;

Studies confirming the Virus Killing Effectiveness of Mixing Sodium Chlorite with Citric Acid
Sodium Chlorite with Citric Acid is approved by the FDA to spray on food [8] [9] [10].

Further Reading
The Effect of Sodium Hypochlorite and Citric Acid Solutions on Healing of Periodontal Pockets. E M Vieira et al. Feb 1982

The Bactericidal Effects of an Acidified Sodium Chlorite-Containing Oral Moisturizing Gel: A Pilot Study. Iwao Kuroyama et al. Dec 2013.

Effect of Sodium Chloride and Citric Acid on Growth and Toxin Production by A. Caviae and A. Sobria at Moderate and Low Temperatures. B M Abu-Ghazaleh et a. Oct 2000.

Oral Ingestion of Diluted Chlorine Dioxide
There is considerable controversy regarding ingesting a few drops of Chlorine Dioxide that has been diluted in a cup of water. While there exist numerous online testimonials regarding the healing benefits, the FDA has reported that it has received reports of people having

adverse reactions from adding a few drops of Chlorine Dioxide to water.

Toxicity

In studies conducted on rats, Chlorine dioxide was toxic when administered in solution by a single oral dose to rats; at 40 and 80 mg/kg body weight (*this is an extremely high amount*). The animals showed signs of corrosive activity in the stomach and gastrointestinal tract. The calculated oral LD50 was 94 mg/kg body weight. (*Note by Author - Hence Excessive use of Chlorine Dioxide appears to exhibit acidic PH effects upon the body*) [11].

Physical Reactions to Chlorine Dioxide

A research study titled: *Controlled clinical evaluations of chlorine dioxide, chlorite and chlorate in man* that was conducted by J R Lubbers and colleagues, concluded that chlorine dioxide diluted in water was well tolerated when the participants took it consecutively for 12 weeks. What is most interesting in this study is that the researchers found that certain types of people are more sensitive to diluted chlorine dioxide in water than other people. These people were designated to have low level of glucose-6-phosphate dehydrogenase, which makes them more susceptible to oxidative stress.

Further Reading

FDA Sponsors Study pilot program for a Generally Recognized as safe (GRAS) determination for the safe use of chlorine dioxide generated by the notifier's PureMash system in the production of food grade and non-food grade ethanol.

A study involving groups of 10 male and 10 female Sprague-Dawley rats received approximately 0, 2, 4, 6, or 12 mg/kg body weight per day and 0, 2, 5, 8, or 15 mg/kg body weight per day, respectively, of aqueous chlorine dioxide in drinking-water for 90 days (*Daniel et al., 1990*). There were no treatment-related deaths or clinical signs of toxicity. There were reductions in body weight gain and food consumption at the highest exposure level [12].

How to Make Chlorine Dioxide
A simple form of Chlorine Dioxide can be made at home by combining sodium chlorite powder with citric acid (*from lemons*). Just a few drops of this solution are than added to a cup of distilled water. Although I am not going to publish the formula here, I urge the reader to find a respectable website (how to make Miracle Mineral Solution) to find the proper ratio and amounts needed and to remember that the full strength drops must be completely diluted in a cup of water if one wants to try it orally.

Concluding Summary
While a pharmaceutical COVID-19 vaccine may eventually become available, it could take years to perfect and there are already millions of people in the United States who avoid the flu vaccine due to religious reasons. Also a vaccine can have serious side effects. Chlorine Dioxide, when properly diluted with water, shows minimal side effects. Not one single death of anyone dying from taking chlorine dioxide diluted in water has ever been reported in the scientific medical literature.

Further Reading
Investigation on virucidal activity of chlorine dioxide. experimental data on feline calicivirus, HAV and Coxsackie B. R Zoni. et al. Sept 2007. This study showed COMPLETE

INACTIVATION of the virus by Chlorine Dioxide and that its effects are DOSE DEPENDENT.

Study on the resistance of severe acute respiratory syndrome-associated coronavirus. Xin-Wei Wang et al. March 2005.

A comparison of the virucidal properties of chlorine, chlorine dioxide, bromine chloride and iodine. Taylor, G.R., Butler, M., 1982b. J. Hyg. (Lond.) 89, 321–328.

Numbered References. Chapter 12

(1) Satomura K, Kitamura T, Kawamura T, Shimbo T, Watanabe M, Kamei M, et al. Great cold investigators:
prevention of upper respiratory tract infections by gargling. A randomized trial. Am J PrevMed 2005; 29:
302-7, https://doi.org/10.1016/j.amepre.2005.06.013.

(1a) Ogata N, Shibata T. Effect of chlorine dioxide gas of extremely low concentration on absenteeism of
schoolchildren. Int J Med Med Sci 2009; 1(7): 288-9.

(2) Dental Tribune - Clinical use of Chlorine dioxide in the prevention of Coronavirus spread through dental aerosols. May 24, 2020.

(3) Multicomponent spectroscopic investigations of salivary antioxidant consumption by an oral rinse preparation containing the stable free radical species chlorine dioxide (ClO2).Lynch E., et al.

(3a) Lubbers JR, Chauan SR, Bianchine JR. Controlled clinical evaluations of chlorine dioxide, chlorite and
chlorate in man. Environ Health Perspect 1982; 46: 57-62, https://doi.org/10.1289/ehp.824657.

(4) Firms fined £350,000 for chlorine dioxide death. BBC News.

(5) Chlorine Gas Inhalation Human Clinical Evidence of Toxicity and Experience in Animal Models Carl W. White and James G. Martin. July 2010.

(6) Chlorine Gas for the Prevention of Infectious Diseases. Norio Ogata. R and D Center.

(7) Protective effect of low-concentration chlorine dioxide gas against influenza A virus infection. Norio Ogata et al. J Gen Virol. 2008 Jan;89(Pt 1):60-67. doi: 10.1099/vir.0.83393-0.

(8) Efficacy of Sodium Hypochlorite and Acidified Sodium Chlorite in Preventing Browning and Microbial Growth on Fresh-Cut Produce. Shih Hui Sun. et al. Sept 2012.

(9) A combination of Sodium Chlorite with Citric Acid and Trisodium Phosphate has been found to reduce Pathogenic bacteria on refrigerated chicken.

(10) Effectiveness of Trisodium Phosphate, Acidified Sodium Chlorite, Citric Acid, and Peroxyacids Against Pathogenic Bacteria on Poultry During Refrigerated Storage. Elena del Río et al. Sept 2007.

(11) Concise International Chemical Assessment Document 37. World Health Organization.

(12) Concise International Chemical Assessment Document 37. World Health Organization.

Chapter 13. The Powerful Healing of the Natural Antibiotic Ajwain.

Over the years of after having written thousands of pages about anti-aging, one trend stands out; some of the most powerful anti-aging substances are antibiotics. So when my research turned up Ajwain, I decided to combine it with the St. Germain Extract, which is also a very mild natural antibiotic. The St. Germain formula surfaced during the 1700's which was a time where Alchemy was popular. To my surprise I discovered that it has a very powerful anti-aging effect, as well as antiviral and anti-microbial. Indeed after further research and study I discovered that Ajwain is stronger than some antibiotics. For example, a research study found that Ajwain is abundant in Thymol, which has been shown to kill bacteria resistant microorganisms and shows effectiveness against third generation antibiotics as well as multi-drug resistant microbial pathogens. The study found that Ajwain works as a natural plant based 4th generation herbal antibiotic formulation [1].

Anti-malarials are some of the most potent weapons one can use to fight COVID-19. Ajwain exhibits anti-malarial properties; hence an anti-malarial may hold promise in the field of anti-aging regenerative medicine in the future.

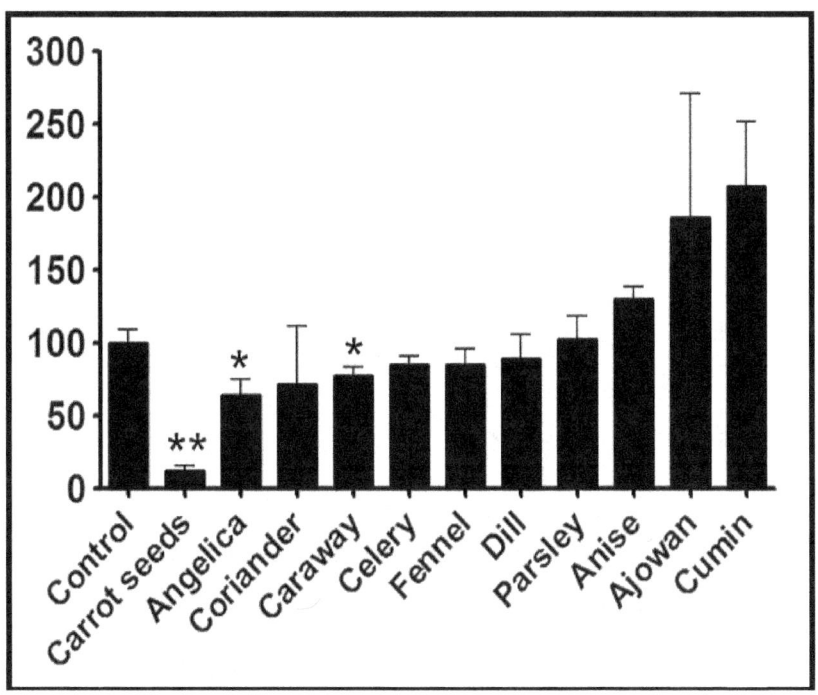

The above image shows that Ajwain extract (*and cumin*) exhibits powerful protection against DNA damage. The synergy that occurs with Ajwain and the St. Germain formula may be due to the fact that the St. Germain formula contains Anise. The above study also stated that Ajwain shows significant free radical scavenging activity and that Ajwain extract exhibited the highest antioxidant activity, followed by carrot seed extract [2]. This is an interesting finding because carrot extract synergizes very well with St. Germain Tea, but for some reason not with the extract of St. Germain.

My Personal Experiences Using Ajwain
From my personal experience of purchasing Ajwain seeds and making them into an extract, I have discovered that it keeps for months on end, as does the St. Germain Extract.

This is a key attribute to an anti-aging compound, in that it does not spoil easily. Many extracts I have made over the years go bad within a few months or sometimes weeks, but I discovered that the most potent anti-aging extracts would last for years. You can find out how to make your own extracts in my book The Official Guidebook of How to Make Tinctures and Alchemy Spagyric Formulas. The majority of Ajwain I purchase has been from India which currently seems to be short supply; perhaps to greater awareness that Ajwain is an effective natural antibiotic and people are using it as a preventative against COVID-19. Now let's get down to understanding why Ajwain is such a powerful natural antibiotic.

Why Ajwain is a Powerful Natural Antibiotic
Research conducted by A. Luca and colleagues at King Saud University, published in the Arabian Journal of Chemistry, under the heading Diverse biological effects of the essential oil from Iranian Trachyspermum ammi in 2016, that the oil of Ajwain exhibited antibacterial activity that was comparable to that of the prescribed antibiotic ciprofloxacin. The researchers identified the major constituent as thymol which was present at a remarkable 67.4% in the oil [3].

Thymol is found in abundance in the spice Thyme, which has powerful natural anti-microbial properties (*as does the spice oregano*). Many anti-microbials are used to preserve food and indeed Ajwain has been proven to protect against food spoilage by inhibiting the growth of all test fungi by a remarkable 72-90%. This is a remarkable finding.

The study goes on to state that Ajwain essential oil killed Gram-positive bacteria (*which in the mouth causes tooth decay*) and that it was quite effective in doing so; with S. aureus being more susceptible to the Ajwain oil than E. faecalis. As I show in my book The Complete Guide to Natural Toothache Remedies and Re-mineralization, S.

aureus is partly responsible for tooth decay; hence an Ajwain mouthwash may help prevent cavities; some mouthwashes already have thymol or thyme in them. Further studies need to confirm this hypothesis.

The researchers in the study also stated Ajwain exhibited significant radical scavenging activity and also shows major antioxidant potential. This has been confirmed by earlier studies (*Alma et al., 2003; Ozturk, 2012; Quiroga et al., 2015*). This is a major finding because it bumps Ajwain up into the class of anti-aging herbs, due to its extremely high free radical scavenging ability. The study also concluded that Ajwain's antioxidant activity is comparable to commercially available antioxidants found on the market today. In the same study, in a detailed analysis of Ajwain, researchers found Ajwain oil was as potent in fighting disease causing bacteria with inhibition zones measuring higher than those of a standard antibiotic. The results were especially remarkable for its ability to fight Staphylococcus aureus and Candida albicans, which are found in the stomach, making it a great way to keep the stomach strong and healthy. As a matter of fact, Ajwain has been officially administered to treat or cure stomach disorders [4] [5].

Ajwain Effectively Kills numerous types of Colon Cancer Cells

Colon cancer comes in many types and varieties, making it hard to treat. The same study [5] discovered to the authors' amazement that Ajwain oil was particularly cytotoxic on colon carcinoma cells (*it kills colon cancer cells*) and was active against ALL OF THEM. The results were also dose dependant, meaning a "*sweet spot*" exists that the right dosage must be taken in order to properly kill all the colon cancer cells. The study also discovered that Ajwain oil was effective in killing breast cancer cells (MDA-MB 231) and melanoma (A375). The researchers also stated that Ajwain oil also exhibited strong cytotoxic activity on colon cancer cells which was trigged by an enhancement of immune system cells, suggesting that Ajwain oil also creates a strong and robust immune system.

The Healing Power of Thymol
Thymol is found in abundance in the cooking spice Thyme (*it also contains c-terpinene*). It is found in Ajwain at levels ranging from 35% to 60%. Thymol is a strong natural germicide, fungicide and antispasmodic agent. The non-thymol constituents in Ajwain oil are made up of c-terpinene, a-pinene, b-pinene, p-cymene and other minor components (*Zarshenas et al., 2014*). Because its anti-microbial properties are so concentrated, it is key that it is properly processed and the dosages used are properly administered for maximum healing. Thymol has been shown to be effective in killing lung cancer cells (*Ozkan and Erdogan, 2012*), leukemia cells and human glioblastoma cells (*Hsu et al., 2011*). Studies by Bourgou et al. (*2010*) looked at the cytotoxic activity of c-terpinene and its effectiveness against human lung cancer cells and colon cancer cells achieving a remarkable IC50 P 100 lM (13.62 lg/mL) on both cell lines.

Ajwain Oil is Fungi Toxic
Various form of mold/fungi can be or turn toxic. Ajwain essential oil has been shown to be effective across a broad spectrum of fungi toxic fungi such as A. niger, A. ochraceus, P. viridicatum, P. madriti, F. monoliforme, F. graminearum, Pencillium citrium, A. flavus, A. oryzae and C. Lunata [6].

Anti-Malarial Potential of Ajwain Oil

Ajwain oil has been scientifically validated to exhibit repellent type activity against the effects of the mosquito Anopheles stephensi (*Pandey et al., 2009*) and Ajwain oil exhibited larvicidal activity against Aedes aegypti (*Seo et al., 2012*). This makes it a promising treatment for the management of malaria and yellow fever caused by mosquitoes.

Ajwain oil as a Male Contraceptive

Ajwain oil shows strong spermicidal potential, making it a possible effective substance for use as a natural male contraceptive (*Paul and Kang, 2011, 2012*). This may mean that excessive use of Ajwain may cause temporary sterility, although further research is needed to confirm this hypothesis.

A Detailed Scientific Analysis of Ajwain Seed

Besides Thymol, Ajwain seed is made up of the following [7] -

fiber (11.9%)
carbohydrates (38.6%)
tannins, glycosides, moisture (8.9%)
protein (15.4%)
fat (18.1%)
saponins, flavone and mineral matter (7.1%)

It also contains calcium, phosphorous, iron and nicotinic acid.

The fruit of Ajwain contains a 2% to 4% brownish essential oil, with thymol being the major constituent (35% to 60%)

In the nonthymol fraction analysis Ajwain contains -

para-cymene, γ-terpenine, dipentene, α-terpinene, α- and β-pinenes and carvacrol. Small amounts of myrcene, camphene and α-3-carene have also been found in the plant Ajwain. When Ajwain is made into an alcoholic extract, it exhibits strong hygroscopic saponin properties [8] [9].

This is an important finding, because as I illustrate in great detail throughout my anti-aging books, substances that exhibit hygroscopic properties reduce bad bacteria's ability to cling to surfaces. They are especially effective in preventing tooth decay as I outline in detail in my natural tooth healing remedies book shown earlier.

When it comes to the concentrated oil content in Ajwain, the main oils in Ajwain are carvone (46%), limonene (38%), and dillapiole (9%). This means that Ajwain may exhibit synergy with Rosemary, which also contains an abundance of Carvone. Further studies are needed to confirm this hypothesis. Carvone is also very effective in helping to reduce coughs when made into an aerosol spray or inhaled [10] [11].

The Detoxification Properties of Ajwain
Ajwain has been shown to be effective in the detoxification of aflatoxins [12].

And remarkably Ajwain was shown to protect the liver against toxins. The hepatoprotective actions (*in vivo*) exhibited a remarkable 80% protective effect in studies conducted on mice when they were injected with paracetamol, at lethal doses (1 g/kg) to stimulate liver damage. Ajwain was shown to normalize high serum levels of liver enzymes which caused liver damage from injecting the paracetamol into the mice. In short summary, Ajwain protected the liver from damage [13].

Ajwain Protects Against Oxidative Stress

When oxidative stress was induced in rats (*one of the primarily cause of aging and disease*), when the rats were fed Ajwain extract before hand, it resulted in increased levels of their superoxide dismutase, catalase and glutathione levels. The study concluded that the rats taking Ajwain extract before experiencing oxidative stress, that the Ajwain extract protected them against the effects of oxidative stress. This is a significant finding because oxidative stress can occur during and after extreme exercise. This means taking an extract of Ajwain before or after extreme exercise may help a person recover faster and / or increase their stamina and endurance [14].

Ajwain Enhances Bile Acids and Increases Digestion

As I show in my latest anti-aging book Reverse Aging Naturally. Alchemy and Ayurveda Longevity Anti-aging Secrets., healthy bile acids are vital to a long lifespan. Researchers studying the digestive stimulant properties (*in vivo and in vitro*) of Ajwain discovered that it increased the secretion of gastric acid (*which is a healthy bile acid*). The study further goes on to state that the levels of Gastric acid increased almost nearly four-fold by Ajwain. This is a major finding because as the body ages, it secretes less bile acids, making it harder for the stomach to effectively pass food through the stomach [15].

In studies conducted on rats, adding Ajwain to their diet reduced the amount of time food passed through their stomachs and most of all it enhanced the activity of their digestive enzymes and caused a higher secretion of bile acids to be secreted. This also is a major finding because a strong healthy digestive system is one of the 5 golden keys to longevity [16].

Ajwain Lowers lipids

Another hallmark of aging are lipids. When Ajwain powder was added at the dose of 2 g/kg per body weight, it was found to be extensively effective in lowering lipids via decreased cholesterol levels [17].

Ajwain Boosts Estrogen

Many ingredients listed in the St. Germain Formula are shown to boost Estrogen Levels. This in turn strengthens bones. A research study conducted by The National Dairy Research Institute in India investigated the estrogenic content of some herbs, including Ajwain's ability to increase milk yield in dairy cattle. Out of a number of 8 herbs that were tested for total phytoestrogen content, Ajwain came in second (473 ppm) making it a powerful Estrogen booster (*total phytoestrogen contents 131-593 ppm*) [18].

Ajwain's Anti-inflammatory Effects

Inflammation is one of the hallmarks of aging. It reduces the body's ability to fight off disease and it reduces the body's ability to recover from injury. In studies conducted on animals, Ajwain exhibited significant ($P<0.001$) anti-inflammatory effects due to its ability to increase the size of their adrenal glands and extracts of Ajwain Seeds exhibited significant anti-inflammatory properties [19].

Further Reading

Diverse biological effects of the essential oil from Iranian Trachyspermum ammi. Luca A et al. King Saud University. Arabian Journal of Chemistry. 2016.

Chemical constituents, antifungal and anti-oxidative effects of Ajwain essential oil and its acetone extract. Singh G., Maurya S., Catalan C., de Lampasona M.P. J. Agric. Food Chem. 2004;52:3292-3296. doi: 10.1021/jf035211c.

Numbered References. Chapter 13

(1) Saxena AP, Vyas KM. Antimicrobial activity of seeds of some ethnomedicinal plants. J Econ Taxonomic Bot. 1986;8:291–300.

(2) Potent chemopreventive/antioxidant activity detected in common spices of the Apiaceae family. Jeyaprakash Jeyabalan. et al. Oct 2015.

(3) Saxena AP, Vyas KM. Antimicrobial activity of seeds of some ethnomedicinal plants. J Econ Taxonomic Bot. 1986;8:291–300.

(4) The wealth of India, A dictionary of Indian Raw Materials and Industrial Products Publications and Information Directorate. Vol. 21. New Delhi: CSIR; 1976.

(5) Singh VK, Singh S, Singh DK. Phytochemistry Pharmacology. Vol. 2. Houston, Texas, USA: Stadium Press; 2003. Pharmacological effects of spices. In Recent Progress in Medicinal Plants; pp. 321–53.

(6) Antibacterial and Antifungal Activities of Spices. Qing Liu et al. June 2017.

(7) Ishikawah T, Sega Y, Kitajima J. Water-soluble constituents of ajowan. Chem Pharm Bull. 2001;49:840–4.

(8) Chopra RN. Chopra's Indigenous Drug of India. 2nd ed. Calcutta: Academic Publishers; 1982. pp. 93–4.

(9) Garg SN, Kumar S. A new glucoside from Trachyspermum ammi. Fitoterapia.

(10) Boskabady MH, Jandaghi P, Kiani S, Hasanzadeh L. Antitussive effect of Carum copticum in guinea pigs. J Ethnopharmacol. 2005;97:79–82.

(11) Choudhury S. Composition of the seed oil of Trachyspermum ammi (L.) Sprague from northeast India. J Essent Oil Res. 1998;10:588-90.

(12) Velazhahan R, Vijayanandraj S, Vijayasamundeeswari A, Paranidharan V, Samiyappan R, Iwamoto T, et al. Detoxification of aflatoxins by seed extracts of the medicinal plant, Trachyspermum ammi (L.) Sprague ex Turrill Structural analysis and biological toxicity of degradation product of aflatoxin G1. Food Control. 2010;21:719-25.

(13) Gilani AH, Jabeen Q, Ghayur MN, Janbaz KH, Akhtar MS. Studies on the antihypertensive, antispasmodic, bronchodilator and hepatoprotective activities of the Carum copticum seed extract. Journal of Ethnopharmacol. 2005;98:127-35.

(14) Anilakumar KR, Saritha V, Khanum F, Bawa AS. Ameliorative effect of ajwain extract on hexachlorocyclohexane-induced lipid peroxidation in rat liver. Food Chem Toxicol. 2009;47:279-82.

(15) Vasudevan K, Vembar S, Veeraraghavan K, Haranath PS. Influence of intragastric perfusion of aqueous spice extracts on acid secretion in anesthetized albino rats. Indian J Gastroenterol. 2000;19:53-6.

(16) Platel K, Srinivasan K. Studies on the influence of dietary spices on food transit time in experimental rats. Nutr Res. 2001;21:1309-14.

(17) Javed IM, Akhtar T, Khaliq MZ, Khan G, Muhammad M. Antihyperlipidaemic effect of Trachyspermum ammi (Ajwain) in rabbits. In: Faisalabad: Proc 33rd All Pakistan Science Conference University of Agriculture. 2002:80-1.

(18) Kaur H. Estrogenic activity of some herbal galactogogue constituents. Indian J Anim Nutr. 1998;15:232-4.

(19) Thangam C, Dhananjayan R. Antiinflammatory Potential Of The Seeds Of Carum Copticum Linn. Indian J Pharmacol. 2003;35:388-91. (Trachyspermum ammi. Ranjan Bairwa et al. Jan 2012).

Chapter 14. The Universal Healing Properties of Black Cumin Seed.

One of the more promising natural candidates to defeat COVID-19, Nigella sativa L. - Ranunculaceae (*black cumin seed*) has been shown to possess multifaceted properties due to thymoquinone being effective against H9N2 and cytomegaloviral diseases (*Tavakkoli et al., 2017*). Further research may reveal that the substance thymoquinone, found in black cumin seed, helps defeat COVID-19. Studies also have shown its effectiveness in treating asthma patients (*Koshak et al., 2017*).

A research study titled: *Nigella sativa L as a potential phytotherapy for coronavirus disease 2019: A mini review of in silico studies* that was conducted by Dr Abdulrahman E. Koshak and colleagues in August of 2020 performed a literature search for published between the years 1990 and 2020 (PubMed, Science Direct, Scopus, and Google Scholar) using the search terms Nigella sativa, black seed, coronavirus, SARS-CoV-2, and COVID-19. The results of the search showed that 8 in silico studies showed that some compounds of N sativa, including thymohydroquinone, nigelledine, α-hederin, hederagenin and thymoquinone exhibit high to moderate affinity with SARS-CoV-2 enzymes and proteins. The authors concluded that these substances may inhibit SARS-CoV-2 replication and its attachment to host cell receptors.

Studies have shown clinical benefits in asthma patients. In a double-blind, randomized placebo-controlled study, participants who took soft gel capsules of cold-pressed N. sativa oil (0.7% thymoquinone) showed improved asthma control and a significant improvement in shortness of breath. The study also found a remarkable normalization of blood eosinophilia count (*Koshak et al., 2017*). Also the release of IL-2, IL-6 as well as PGE2 in T-lymphocytes, (and in monocytes) was suppressed.

Now let's explore what Black Cumin Seed is and its numerous healing benefits upon the body.

Black Cumin Seed (*Nigella sativa*) belongs to the Ranunculaceae botanical family of plant species. It flourishes in the Middle East, and is cultivated in Eastern Europe and Western Asia.

Black Cumin Seed is also included in the list of natural substances to treat ill health in Indian traditional medicine, the Tibb-e-Nabavi [1]. The majority of the therapeutic effects experienced by taking Black Cumin Seed come from the substance known as thymoquinone, which is the main bioactive constituent of the oil found in the seeds [2].

Black Cumin exerts powerful protective effects against the liver, kidney, brain, heart and lungs. It also exhibits protection against various toxic agents; either chemical or natural toxins present in the environment [3]. A key finding about Black Cumin is that Like Quercetin (*one of nature's most powerful anti-aging substances*), the thymoquinone in Black Cumin seed exhibits powerful lead chelating abilities [4].

Thymoquinone Protects against methionine induced hyperhomocysteinemia

This is a good thing if you eat lots of spirulina because spirulina contains an abundance of methionine and too much methionine in the diet can be detrimental [5]. Thymoquinone has also been shown in animal studies to protect against excessive levels of Sodium Fluoride [6] [7] [8]. Thymoquinone also protects against Bisphenol A (BPA). BPA is widely used in the resin and plastics industry; being the prime component of plastic bottles such as food, beverage and baby bottles [9].

Black Cumin Protects against Natural Toxins
Black Cumin and its main component Thymoquinone exhibit antidotal effects against some natural toxins including D-galactosamine, mycotoxins and lipopolysaccharides (LPS) [10] [11] [12].

Polysaccharides
Sulfated polysaccharides from red algae (saltwater) exhibited strong antiviral bioactivity shown in a study by Nagle et al. (*2020*). The main constituents responsible for the antiviral activity were chondroitin sulfate and heparin (*Ghosh et al., 2009*). These are potent against several retrovirus (*Talyshinsky et al., 2002*); including HSV-1 and HSV-2 (*Nagle et al., 2020*) etc [12a].

Thymoquinone is one of Nature's Most Powerful Natural Antioxidants
Thymoquinone exerts strong antioxidant properties because of its free radical scavenging ability [13].
Thymoquinone Protects the Brain [14] [15] [16].

Thymoquinone Protects Mammals against Diesel Exhaust Pollution
In a study where mice were given thymoquinone before being exposed to diesel exhaust, their lungs were found to be protected from the diesel fumes after being exposed to the exhaust for 18 hours. Also the antibiotic Cisplatin can aggravate the pulmonary dysfunction produced by diesel exhaust particles. I can imagine the scientists hooking up their car exhaust to a small box with a valve controlling the rate of exhaust into a small box with the mice. The poor mice, at least they survived!! [17].

Black Cumin seed by itself or in combination with dexamethasone, was shown to be equal to the effectiveness of dexamethasone, which is an anti-dote used to treat people exposed to the chemical warfare agent Sulfur mustard [18].

Black Cumin Protects against Indoor Air Pollution

Black Cumin seed also protects against air pollution because the seeds contain an abundance of Thymoquinone. Toluene is an airborne pollutant commonly found in homes and buildings. Studies conducted on rats showed that chronic exposure to Toluene caused severe degeneration in the frontal cortex neurons. However treating the rats with thymoquinone reduced this damage to some degree [19].

Further Reading
Kanter M. Protective effects of thymoquinone on the neuronal injury in frontal cortex after chronic toluene exposure. J. Mol. Histol. 2011;42:39–46.

Black Cumin Reduces the Side Effects of Strong Antibiotics

Black Cumin Seed has shown protective effects against side the effects of the medications Isoniazid, Oxytetracyclin, Amikacin, Gentamicin as well as protecting against the side effects of the anti-cancers Cisplatin, Methotrexate, Cyclophosphamide, Tamoxifen and Imidacloprid. It has also been shown to protect against Carbon tetrachloride and Acetaminophen. The meta study also states that Thymoquinone acts as an antidote against natural toxins. These include mycotoxins and endotoxins and the metals lead, aluminum mercury and cadmium as well as the industrial pesticides, propoxur, fenitrothion, imidacloprid, chlorpyrifos and acetamiprid. It also shows protective effects against the detergents and solvents CCl4, ethanol, toluene and nitrilotriacetate and the environmental industrial pollutant DEP.

Black Cumin Protects against Drug Overdose

The study goes on to state that Thymoquinone and Black Cumin have shown potential to protect the body's tissues against some overdoses of various drugs, immunosuppresents, analgesics anticancer, various antibiotics, antiretroviral and anti-seizure medications.

Black Cumin Oil Exhibits Synergy with Vitamin C

The study also showed that in experiments involving liver and kidney inflammation that was caused by an overdose of the antibiotic Oxytetracyclin, that a combination of Black Cumin Oil and Vitamin C restored healthy liver functioning in experiments with rabbits and that Thymoquinone has also been shown to protect against the fungus aflatoxins and Verrucarin J.

Black Cumin Seed has also exerted synergism with human parathyroid hormone. This hormone is used to improve bone mass, strength and connectivity.

Black Cumin Seed with Echinacea exhibits synergy

A combination of Black Cumin (nigelia Sativa) and Echinacea given to animals was shown enhance their immune system as well as improve their antioxidant status [20].

Summary

Like Berberine's multifaceted healing properties, Black Cumin seed exhibits a broad spectrum of protective activities against toxins found in our environment; manmade or natural. Hence, berberine may show some of the same protective properties as Black Cumin Seed and versa. Black Cumin Seed is highly recommended for those living in regions where environmental toxins are at above average levels.

A scientific analysis of Black Cumin Seed Oil (30%-45%; oleic and linoleic acids), triterpenoids, saponins; essential oil, a high concentration of thymoquinone (2-isopropyl-5-methyl-1,4-benzoquinone), (*Lutterodt et al., 2010*). Note the thymoquinone in Black Cumin seed is not found in large concentrations in aqueous preparations of Black Cumin Seed [21].

Recommended Dosage
Taken with a fatty oil for best absorption. The essential oil may also offer relief. I personally take 1 teaspoon of black cumin seeds mixed in half a cup of water.

Further Reading
Nagi MN, Alam K, Badary OA, Al-Shabanah OA, Al-Sawaf HA, Al-Bekairi AM. Thymoquinone protects against carbon tetrachloride hepatotoxicity in mice via an antioxidant mechanism. Biochem. Mol. Biol. Int. 1999;47:153-9.

Korany NS, Ezzat BA. Prophylactic effect of green tea and Nigella sativa extracts against fenitrothion-induced toxicity in rat parotid gland. Arch. Oral. Biol. 2011;56:1339-46).

Koka P, Mondal D, Schultz M, Abdel-Mageed A, Agrawal K. Studies on molecular mechanisms of growth inhibitory effects of thymoquinone against prostate cancer cells: role of reactive oxygen species. Exp. Biol. Med. 2010;235:751-60.

Hosseinzadeh H, Parvardeh S, Nassiri-Asl M, Mansouri M-T. Intracerebroventricular administration of thymoquinone, the major constituent of Nigella sativa seeds, suppresses epileptic seizures in rats. Med. Sci. Monitor. 2005;11:BR106-BR10.

Suddek GM. Protective role of thymoquinone against liver damage induced by tamoxifen in female rats. Canadian J. Physiol. Pharmacol. 2014;92:640-4.

Thymoquinone therapy abrogates toxic effect of cadmium on rat testes. Andrologia. 2015;47:417-26.Toxicol. Pathol.

2014;66:13-7.

Mabrouk A, Ben Cheikh H. Thymoquinone supplementation reverses lead-induced oxidative stress in adult rat testes. Gen. Physiol. Biophys. 2015;34:65-72.

Numbered Referrences. Chapter 14

(1) The medicine of Prophet Mohammad), Unani Tebb, and (Rajsekhar S, Kuldeep B. Pharmacognosy and pharmacology of Nigella sativa- A review. Int. Res. J. Pharm. 2011;2:36–9.

(2) (Black Seed (Nigella Sativa) and its Constituent Thymoquinone as an Antidote or a Protective Agent Against Natural or Chemical Toxicities. Alireza Tavakkoli et al. Dec 2017.

(3) Black Seed (Nigella Sativa) and its Constituent Thymoquinone as an Antidote or a Protective Agent Against Natural or Chemical Toxicities. Alireza Tavakkoli et al. Dec 2017.

(4) Radad K, Hassanein K, Al-Shraim M, Moldzio R, Rausch WD. Thymoquinone ameliorates lead-induced brain damage in Sprague Dawley rats. Exp. Fouad AA, Jresat I.

(5) El-Saleh SC, Al-Sagair OA, Al-Khalaf MI. Thymoquinone and Nigella sativa oil protection against methionine-induced hyperhomocysteinemia in rats. Int. J. Cardiol. 2004;93:19–23.

(6) Blaszczyk I, Birkner E, Kasperczyk S. Influence of methionine on toxicity of fluoride in the liver of rats. Biol.Trace Elem. Res. 2011;139:325–31,

(7) Nabavi SM, Nabavi SF, Eslami S, Moghaddam AH. In-vivo protective effects of quercetin against sodium fluoride-induced oxidative stress in the hepatic tissue. Food Chem. 2012;132:931–5.

(8) Abdel-Wahab WM. Protective effect of thymoquinone on sodium fluoride-induced hepatotoxicity and oxidative stress in rats. J. Basic Appl. Zool. 2013;66:263–70.

(9) (Abdel-Wahab WM. Thymoquinone attenuates toxicity and oxidative stress induced by bisphenol A in liver of male rats. Pakistan J. Biol. Sci. 2014;17:1152–60.

(10) (Nili-Ahmadabadi A, Tavakoli F, Hasanzadeh G, Rahimi H, Sabzevari O. Protective effect of pretreatment with thymoquinone against Aflatoxin B(1) induced liver toxicity in mice. Daru. 2011;19:282-7), (Abdel-Wahhab MA, Aly SE. Antioxidant property of Nigella sativa (black cumin) and Syzygium aromaticum in rats during aflatoxicosis. J. Appl. Toxicol. 2005;25:218-23.

(11) Mohamed saleem Gani A, Ahmed John S. Evalution of hepatoprotective effect of Nigella sativa L. Int. J. Pharm. Pharm. Sci. 2013;5:428-30.

(12) Thymoquinone supplementation ameliorates acute endotoxemia-induced liver dysfunction in rats. Pakistan J. Pharm. Sci. 2010;23:131-7.

(12a) Herbal immune-boosters: Substantial warriors of pandemic Covid-19 battle. Kanika Khannaa et al. Sept 2020.

(13) Hosseinzadeh H, Parvardeh S, Asl MN, Sadeghnia HR, Ziaee T. Effect of thymoquinone and Nigella sativa seeds oil on lipid peroxidation level during global cerebral ischemia-reperfusion injury in rat hippocampus. Phytomedicine. 2007;14:621-7.

(14) Hosseinzadeh H, Parvardeh S, Nassiri-Asl M, Mansouri M-T. Intracerebroventricular administration of thymoquinone, the major constituent of Nigella sativa seeds, suppresses epileptic seizures in rats. Med. Sci. Monitor. 2005;11:BR106-BR10).

(15) Parvardeh S, Nassiri-Asl M, Mansouri MT, Hosseinzadeh H. Study on the anticonvulsant activity of thymoquinone, the major constituent of Nigella sativa L seeds, through intracerebroventricular injection. J. Med. Plants. 2005;4:45-52.

(16) Mehri S, Shahi M, Razavi BM, Hassani FV, Hosseinzadeh H. Neuroprotective effect of thymoquinone in acrylamide induced neurotoxicity in wistar rats. Iran. J. Basic Med. Sci. 2014;17:1007-1011.

(17) Nemmar A, Al-Salam S, Zia S, Marzouqi F, Al-Dhaheri A, Subramaniyan D. Contrasting actions of diesel exhaust particles on the pulmonary and cardiovascular systems and the effects of thymoquinone. Br. J. Pharmacol. 2011;164:1871–82), (Ali BH, Al Za'abi M, Shalaby A, Manoj P, Waly MI, Yasin J. The effect of thymoquinone treatment on the combined renal and pulmonary toxicity of cisplatin and diesel exhaust particles. Exp. Biol. Med. 2015;240:1698–707.

(18) Boskabady MH, Vahedi N, Amery S, Khakzad MR. The effect of Nigella sativa alone, and in combination with dexamethasone, on tracheal muscle responsiveness and lung inflammation in sulfur mustard exposed guinea pigs. J. Ethnopharmacol. 2011;137:1028–34.

(19) Black Seed (Nigella Sativa) and its Constituent Thymoquinone as an Antidote or a Protective Agent Against Natural or Chemical Toxicities. Alireza Tavakkoli et al. Dec 2017.

(20) Comparative immune response and pathogenicity of the H9N2 avian influenza virus after administration of Immulant ®, based on Echinacea and Nigella sativa, in stressed chickens. Abdelfattah H Eladl et al. May 2019.

(21) COVID-19: Is There Evidence for the Use of Herbal Medicines as Adjuvant Symptomatic Therapy? Daˆ maris Silveira et al. September 2020.

Chapter 15. Immune System Boosting Nutraceutical Formulas You can Make at Home.

Foeniculum vulgare Mill.
Foeniculum is used for coughs associated with cold and fever (*EMA, 2007; WHO, 2007*). An ethanol extract or the essential oil of F. vulgare was shown to exhibit antiinflammatory and analgesic activity in rats (*Tanira et al., 1996; Özbek, 2005; Him et al., 2008; Araujo et al., 2013; Elizabeth et al., 2014*).

In a evidence-based analysis, eighteen phytotherapeutic preparations were stated to have a role in the management of viral respiratory diseases, exhibiting various levels of immunological responses (*Portella et al., 2020*). The four herbs stated in the study were - [Echinacea purpurea (L.) Moench, Scutellaria baicalensis Georgi] and Glycyrrhiza glabra L.,Sambucus nigra L.

Echinacea
Preclinical evidence showing enhanced production of immune cells using Sambucus nigra L., polysaccharide-rich extracts from Echinacea, medicinal mushrooms, and Larch (Larix sp.) arabinogalactans-rich extracts as well as plant extracts or food supplements that show an abundance of Vitamin D (*Alschuler et al., 2020*).

Giloy Herbal Extract
Studies on Giloy herbal extract showed it may enhance the immune system (by boosting IgG antibodies) (*Fortunatov, 1952*) and affect humoral immunity and cell regulated immunity (*Winston and Maimes, 2007*).

These next formulas are from my own research and have yet to be verified in research studies. However I have assembled and used these formulas over the years and obtained the information from writing thousands of pages on anti-aging.

The Black Cumin Exercise Recovery Formula
It is a fact that excess exercise stresses the immune system and can make one more susceptible to viral infections. This natural immune system formula is very powerful and should only be taken up to 4 days in a row, than a 3 day break. Use this formula if you want to experience rapid building of new muscle, tissue and strength.

In 1/2 cup of water, add 1 teaspoon of Black Cumin Seed, a pinch of Ginger and allow to soak a minimum of 3 hours.
Next add 1/2 carnosine capsule to the water and stir until dissolved.

Next take the following supplements while drinking the water -

1 Vitamin C capsule
½ capsule of Carnosine
3 drops of Black Cumin Seed Extract (*optional*)
1 1/2 selenium tablet

For an added boost, 30 minutes before taking the above formula take -
6 drops of Cordyceps extract
7 drops of Rhodioa Rosea extract

1 to 2 handfuls of raw walnuts that have had a small amount of grape seed extract added (*which can be found in grape seed extract supplements. Just open the capsule, pour out the powdered extract and make an extract*).

Optional-A handful of 70% Cacao bits. These I get from a health food store in the baking chocolate aisle. They are small M&M sized cacao chocolate pieces. Cacao has been shown to be good for HRV.

Taking Roobios Tea 30 minutes before also synergizes and provides an added boost to the Black Cumin Exercise Recovery Formula.

A combination of Rhodiola Rosea and Cordyceps sinensis was found to enhance aerobic exercise capacity during 2-weeks of high altitude training.

Reference
Rhodiola crenulata- and Cordyceps sinensis-Based Supplement Boosts Aerobic Exercise Performance after Short-Term High Altitude Training. Chung-Yu Chen et al. 2013. HIGH ALTITUDE MEDICINE & BIOLOGY. Volume 15, Number 3, 2014.

The beneficial properties of Salacia Reticulata
Because the majority of the body's immune system is in the stomach, herbs that keep the stomach in good health can be of great advantage. A study decided to take a look at an extract of Salacia Reticulata and its effects upon the body. The study enrolled a group of healthy males aged between 50 and 60 years of age with mildly reduced immunity, and after giving them Salacia Reticulata, found that it induced changes in their intestinal microbiota, improved their T-cell

proliferation index as well as other immunological indices which decline with age. Good sleep has been shown to balance the hormonal responses within the body which helps enhance the body's T-cells (*Calder et al., 2020*). The study also stated that Salacia Reticulata elevated expression levels of their immune-relevant genes. The study came to the conclusion that Salacia Reticulata positively changes the gene expression of a person's peripheral blood cells and the proportion of intestinal microbiota, shifting it towards a younger phenotype. In simple summary, it enhanced the body's immune system which is weekend as one ages. This makes sense because the majority of the body's immune system is located in the stomach (*The stomach in health and disease. R H Hunt, et al. Sept 2015*).

Reference
Improvement in Human Immune Function with Changes in Intestinal Microbiota by Salaciareticulata Extract Ingestion: A Randomized Placebo-Controlled Trial. Yuriko Oda et al. Dec 2015.

The Yogurt Mix Formula
From my book: Living Healthy Beyond 120, A Centurion's Plan for Longevity.

Probiotics Enhances the Immune System of the Elderly
Akatsu et al. (*2013*) showed supplementation with Bifidobacterium longum (found in some yogurt or supplements) helped boost their immune systems (*Herbal immune-boosters: Substantial warriors of pandemic Covid-19 battle. Kanika Khannaa et al. Sept 2020*). Other studies have shown that a wide range of nutraceuticals, probiotics

and herbs are effective against viral infestations as well as help enhance the body's immune system (*Kang et al., 2013; Mousa, 2017*).

Vaccine and Probiotics Synergy
Studies by Bunout et al. (*2002*) showed probiotics improved the immune system in elderly people who were vaccinated. Their antibody production against the influenza B virus was shown to be significantly elevated.

This next formula I am about to share with you is an excellent detox formulation that is mixed into yogurt and eaten in the late afternoon. It also increases the probiotics in the yogurt, contributing to a strong immune system and healthy digestive system.

1/2 Alpha Lipoic Acid & N Acetyl Cysteine Capsule (*or 1/4 Teaspoon*)
1/2 Teaspoon of Cumin Seed
2 Teaspoons of Jigoulan Herb
1 Teaspoon of Cinnamon Powder
1/2 Teaspoon of Astragalus
200 mg of Vitamin B6
1 Now Foods Clinical GI Probiotic Capsule. These capsules contain the probiotic HN019, proven to enhance the immune system in older people

Reference
The Effect of Bifidobacteriumanimalis ssp. lactis HN019 on Cellular Immune Function in Healthy Elderly Subjects: Systematic Review and Meta-Analysis. Miller LE. Et al. Feb 2017.

How to Make The St. Germain Formula
A powerful way to thoroughly clean the colon. A clean colon sets the precedent for long-term lasting health. This formula will also immediately remove constipation and improve digestion as well as heal the eyes.

Uses of St. Germain

Powerful Flu Resistance (when combined with Ajwain)
Enhanced Bone Strength
Immediate relief of Constipation
Removing Dampness (*TCM term*)
Cleansing and Strengthening the Lungs

Take the St. Germain Tea form every 3 to 4 days to enhance sleep and reduce insomnia. The St. Germain formula was developed by count St. Germain, who reputedly had lived a very, very longtime. It is interesting to note that a scientific study conducted on the St. Germain formula (*Fernanda Bastosde MELLO et al. 2006& Paulo D Picon et al. April 2010*) showed it created an increase in white blood cells. (*Pere-Joan Cardona. Aug 2011*). And if you research this further, elderberry, which is used in the St. Germain formula, when elderberry is mixed with Astragalus (*Hanne Frøkiær et al. Oct 2012*) (*which also boosts white blood cells*) it enhances L. acidophilus, which is a probiotic type bacteria found in yogurt. L. acidophilus has also been shown to reduce cavities. This is because Streptococcus mutans, which causes tooth decay (*W J Loesche. Dec 1986*), which is found in the brands of yogurt that contain Acidophilus such as Chobani and Dannon, reduce the chance for one to get cavities due to the L. acidophilus in the yogurt (*Bafna HP et al. 2018*).The formula can also be made into an extract or a tea. If making into an extract you will need to grind up the Star Anise and Fennel Seed.

Removes Damp Heat
If any of you are familiar with Traditional Chinese Medicine (TCM), you will know that dampness is one of the major causes of disease, especially toothache. Toothache is the result of damp heat from stomach yin deficiency. The St. Germain formula, from my experience has been found to greatly strengthen the gums, as well as offer powerful tooth protection against decay. This is because the St. Germain formula is a powerful remover of damp.
You will need –

3 Parts Senna
1.5 Parts Elderberry
1 Part Fennel Seed (*after crushing into a fine powder, slightly more is added to the final formula*)
0.5 Part Star Anise

You will need a lot of Senna because as it is heated and ground up, it will become greatly reduced in size, as the powder becomes extremely very fine.

In a pot with medium heat add the ground up Senna. Next using a fine mist sprayer, spray the Senna and then gently apply a light coating of Cream of Tartar Powder over the Senna and rotate / mix the Senna so the Cream of Tartar is lightly distributed. Apply more mist if needed to thoroughly saturate the Senna, but not too much. Turn the Senna over and over regularly so the Senna does not burn. When the Senna is dry, remove and crush it into a fine powder in a mortar and pestle. It is key that the Senna is dry before doing this or it will be very hard to crush in the mortar and pestle and you will have to send it back to the pot to dry out.

Once you have the Senna powder, measure out the varying parts of the other herbs shown earlier and place in an airtight container. Just be sure to add a little more Senna in the final mix as it becomes extremely fine after crushing.

Usage Instructions
Add between 1 and 1.5 teaspoons to 1 cup of boiling water and let steep for 5 minutes before drinking. The final taste is a liquorice type taste.

The formula will keep for years if stored away from excess heat and light. I have also used an extract that I had kept for over 3 years that was left in a bottle until I ran out of it. The St. Germain formula may have the lasting power of wine, as I have made many extracts over the years and they lose their potency or go bad over time, but the St. Germain extract is one of the rare ones that stands the test of time.

Synergy for the St. Germain Formula.
Before you boil the water add a SLIGHT PINCH of Rosemary Herb and Ginger. Rosemary, like Goji Berry has antioxidants that become stronger with heat and it helps preserve the antioxidants when the St. Germain formula is added to the water later on.

After you have strained the St. Germain Tea add the following for an extra boost -

4 to 6 drops of carrot powder extract
1/2 of 1/2 of 1/3rd of creatine capsule
Take 1 Vitamin D3 capsule (5,000mg)
Take 2 Cod Liver Oil Capsules (1,200mg)

St. Germain Rejuvenation Synergy
Incorporate the St. Germaine formula into your anti-aging diet.

Eat yogurt. Next wait 45 minutes and make a tea out of the St. Germain. As you drink the tea, take 1 reserveratrol capsule, 1,200 mg of cod liver oil and 5,000 mg of D3. Wait another 45 minutes and then take the following –

In a cup of spring water add the following extracts / amounts -
7 drops of elderberry,
2 drops of cayenne pepper,
1 Vitamin C tablet,
4 drops of Astragalus,
3 Tablespoons of honey.

4 to 8 hours later or the following morning, take 1 cup of water with Himalayan salt to restore minerals.

To Remove Excessive Summer Heat Stress
This formula will reduce the energy drain caused by the heat during summer.

In the morning take 1 cup of spring water or other alkaline water and add the following-

2 Drops of Cayenne Pepper Extract
5 Drops of Gingko Extract
A pinch of Himalayan Salt
1 Vitamin C Tablet
1 Vitamin E Tablet

This formula works because Vitamins C and E synergize with one another (*Igarashi O et al. Aug 1991*) and Vitamins C and E also remove heat stress (*Sahin N 2009 et al*). Cayenne pepper is high in both Vitamins C and E (*USDA Nutrient Database*). Ginkgo removes heat stress (*Fuliang Cao et al. 2012*) and Himalayan salt restores minerals lost due to excessive sweat (*Yong-Mei TANG et al. 2016*).

Due to all this synergy, only a small amount is needed and the effects last for up to 4 hours.

Ajwain Extract synergizes very well with St. Germain Extract by adding 8 drops of Ajwain Extract and 4 drops of St. Germain Extract.

The Overnight Rejuven-Essence Formula
From my book: My Book of Stem Cell Longevity Formulas and Nutraceutical AntiAging Combinations.

An excellent formula for boosting the immune system and increasing energy levels and for developing strong and flexible bones; this formula is best taken before going to bed at night with honey. The following morning take the SOD mix mentioned earlier for optimal results. Combine the following and put into capsules:

On a late Friday afternoon or after an especially hard workout, take a food that is high in both niacin and melatonin. For example I use oatmeal seasoned with cinnamon. This is because oatmeal contains adequate levels of both melatonin and niacin. After eating the meal, wait a total of 45 minutes to allow the niacin to fully be absorbed into the body. After 45 minutes have passed, take a food that boosts the body's Superoxide Dismutase levels. I personally take a hot cup of Roobios Tea

(*Aspalathuslinearis*). Physical exercise will also boost your body's Superoxide Dismutase levels (SOD).

Reference
Free radical scavenging ability of Aspalathuslinearis in two in vitro models of diabetes and cancer. Viduranga Y. Waisundaraa and Lee YianHoonb. January 2015.

After another 45 minutes have passed, take the carnosine mix.

The Natural Probiotic Formula
Probioics in yogurt have been shown to enhance the body's immune system. This is a probiotic, but in an extract form. Add a few drops of this formula to plain Greek yogurt that has been mixed with cinnamon and flax seeds to give it an extra boost.

2 drops of Hawthorne Berry Extract
3 drops of Astragalus Extract
5 drops of Salacia Reticulata Extract
3 drops of Elderberry Extract
1 HN109 Probiotic Capsule

Optional -
1/2 Teaspoon of Jigoulan Powder (*or 3 drops of the extract*)
1 Alpha Lipoic Acid Capsule

Chapter 16. Prescription Antibiotics Alter the Healthy Concentration of Stomach Microflora.

In this chapter, I shall explore the effects prescription antibiotics have on the stomach's good bacteria.

Healthy microbiota in the stomach is essential for good health. The best way to maintain this is through eating yogurt, which contains beneficial probiotics, which are packed with nutrients that support the microbiota in our stomach.

After we are born, the microbiota in our stomach rapidly increases in diversity and then reaches an adult-like stage when we turn three. After this, the composition may fluctuate in response to external factors such as antibiotics. Since the introduction of mainstream antibiotics during the 1940s, the short-term effect of pharmaceutically prescribed antibiotics on gut microbiota has been much of a mystery; until now.

Some of the more recent studies looked at the long-term effect of taking prescription antibiotics and discovered that shortly after the person ingests a prescribed antibiotic, that it causes significant alterations to their stomach microbiota. This in turn causes a decrease of between one-fourth to one-third of the microbial diversity in their digestive tract. After the person stops taking the prescribed antibiotic it can take anywhere from several weeks to three months for their gut microbiota to return to healthy levels [1] [2].

Research on animals shows that microbial signals are responsible for the maintenance of healthy lymphocytes, which is important for healthy functioning of the body's immune system (*Suchita Panda et al. Apr 2014*). Other studies show that an absence of healthy stomach microbiota is associated with significant reductions in intestinal levels of neurotransmitters such as GABA and norepinephrine. However these return to normal levels after eating foods that replenish the stomach's microflora (*Suchita Panda et al. Apr 2014*).

SCFA's

These are produced by our colon via anaerobic fermentation of predominantly indigestible dietary carbohydrates and play a key role in the immune system of our body. When mice were fed three of the most popular SCFAs (*butyrate, acetate and propionate*), they alleviated symptoms of depression in the mice [3]. Other studies have discovered a reduced amount of acetate, butyrate and propionate in patients diagnosed with major depression (*Suchita Panda et al. Apr 2014*).

Major Depressive Disorder (MDD) is a psychiatric illness that affects an estimated 300 million people worldwide. It is believed to be responsible for an estimated 800,000 suicide deaths each year (*Stephanie G. Cheung et al. Feb 2019*).

A 2014 research study examined 21 people between the ages of 18 and 80 who were admitted to the hospital for non-digestive diseases (*pneumonia, bacteraemia, bronchitis, urinary tract diseases or prostatitis*). The study found that people who received the broad-spectrum antibiotics β-lactams and fluoroquinolones that the antibiotics decreased the patient's stomach microbiota by 25% regardless of the antibiotic type they were prescribed. It took between 3 to 7 days after the patients first started taking the antibiotics for the reduction in their stomach microbiota to began [4].

Do abnormalities in Healthy Stomach Microflora Contribute to Depression?

Besides the majority of our immune system functioning taking place in our stomachs (*Stephanie G. Cheung et al. Feb 2019*), there exist an estimated four million different genes in the genomes of the gut microbiota. Hence, there exists about 100 to 150 times more genetic information in the human microbiome than the human genome [5].

The job of some of these genes is to perform metabolic functions where they can exert local effects in the gut wall. Alternatively, these microbial metabolites are absorbed and then enter systemic circulation, reaching distant organs, including the brain (*Giorgia Caspani et al. Sept 2019*).

Several studies in humans diagnosed with Major Depression have found differences in their stomach microbiota compared to people not diagnosed with depression [6] [7] [8] [9].

Long term psychological stress has also been shown to alter the composition of the stomach's healthy microbiota [10].

Further Reading
Systematic Review of Gut Microbiota and Major Depression. Stephanie G. Cheung et al. Feb 2019.

Gut microbial metabolites in depression: understanding the biochemical mechanisms. Giorgia Caspani et al. Sept 2019.

Jernberg C, Löfmark S, Edlund C, et al. Long-term impacts of antibiotic exposure on the human intestinal microbiota. Microbiology. 2010;156:3216–23.

Perez-Cobas AE, Artacho A, Knecht H, et al. Differential

effects of antibiotic therapy on the structure and function of human gut microbiota. PLoS One. 2013;8:e80201.

Ng K, Ferreyra J, Higginbottom S, et al. Microbiota-liberated host sugars facilitate post-antibiotic expansion of enteric pathogens. Nature. 2013;502:96-99.

Enhancing the Effectiveness of Antibiotics using Ultrasound
In 2017, antibiotics researchers discovered that low frequency ultrasound waves assisted the strength of antibiotics in both biofilm and planktonic bacteria (*both vitro and in vivo*). The study concluded that low frequency ultrasound promoted the release of antibiotics in an efficient manner and that this enhanced effectiveness may be due to the effect of the ultrasound interacting with antibiotics within the bacterial cells [11].

Further Reading
Carmen J. C., Roeder B. L., Nelson J. L., et al. Treatment of biofilm infections on implants with low-frequency ultrasound and antibiotics. The American Journal of Infection Control. 2005;33(2):78-82. doi: 10.1016/j.ajic.2004.08.002.

Mihai M. M., Holban A. M., Giurcaneanu C., Popa L. G., Oanea R. M., Lazar V. Microbial biofilms: impact on the pathogenesis of periodontitis, cystic fibrosis, chronic wounds and medical device-related infections. Current Topics in Medicinal Chemistry. 2015;15:1552-1576.

Numerical References. Chapter 16.

(1) Dethlefsen L, Huse S, Sogin ML, Relman DA (2008). The pervasive effects of an antibiotic on the human gut microbiota, as revealed by deep 16S rRNA sequencing. PLoS Biol 6: e280.

(2) Jernberg C, Lofmark S, Edlund C, Jansson JK (2007) Long-term ecological impacts of antibiotic administration on the human intestinal microbiota. ISME J 1: 56–66.

(3) Van de Wouw M, Boehme M, Lyte JM, Wiley N, Strain C, O'Sullivan O, Clarke G, Stanton C, Dinan TG, Cryan JF. Short-chain fatty acids: microbial metabolites that alleviate stress-induced brain–gut axis alterations.

(4) Short-Term Effect of Antibiotics on Human Gut Microbiota. Suchita Panda et al. Apr 2014.

(5) Culligan EP, Marchesi JR, Hill C, Sleator RD. Mining the human gut microbiome for novel stress resistance genes. Gut Microbes. 2012;3(4):394–397. doi: 10.4161/gmic.20984.

(6) Exploration of microbiota targets for major depressive disorder and mood related traits. Chung YCE et al.. Psychiatr Res. 2019;111:74–82. doi: 10.1016/j.jpsychires.2019.01.016.

(7) Jiang H et al. Altered fecal microbiota composition in patients with major depressive disorder. Brain Behav Immun. 2015;48:186–194. doi: 10.1016/j.bbi.2015.03.016.

(8) Naseribafrouei A et al. Correlation between the human fecal microbiota and depression. Neurogastroenterol Motil. 2014;26(8):1155–1162. doi: 10.1111/nmo.12378.

(9) (Zheng P et al. Gut microbiome remodeling induces depressive-like behaviors through a pathway mediated by the host's metabolism. Mol Psychiatry. 2016;21(6):786–796. doi: 10.1038/mp.2016.44.

(10) Galley JD, Nelson MC, Yu Z, Dowd SE, Walter J, Kumar PS, Lyte M, Bailey MT. Exposure to a social stressor disrupts the community structure of the colonic mucosa-associated microbiota. BMC Microbiol. 2014;14:189. doi: 10.1186/1471-2180-14-189.

(11) A Review of the Combination Therapy of Low Frequency Ultrasound with Antibiotics. Yun Cai et al. Oct 2017.

Chapter 17. Herbal Energy Supplements You Can Make from Home.

This chapter contains a partial list of my anti-aging formulas included in my anti-aging series of books over the years. Some of these formulas my regular readers will recognize, others have been developed just during the last couple of years as new research has revealed their effectiveness against aging and their supportive roles in physical health, stamina and endurance, and others have been revised.

A July 2020 Study reveals that Exercise Enhances Memory In an article published on July 21st, 2020 on the National Institutes of Health website, titled: *Exercise-induced protein may reverse age-related cognitive decline*, researchers discovered that a protein that is generated during exercise restored loss of memory due to age and that it also generated new brain cell growth in mice.

In studying this protein in adults, older adults displayed more of this protein compared to sedentary adults. The results of this study suggest exercise may exhibit rejuvenating type effects as well as exert preventative effects on aging. The region of the brain that is responsible for rejuvenating brain function due to age related decline during exercise is the hippocampus, as documented in studies conducted on mice. The study found that these proteins existed at higher levels in the blood of the mice that exercised. What is even more interesting is researchers discovered that a protein called GPLD1 was primarily responsible and that this protein is made by the liver.

After discovering this, the researchers than injected the

gene that is responsible for the protein GPLD1 into aged mice, which caused their livers to secrete the protein GPLD1. After a period of three weeks of observation, researchers discovered that the mice exhibited new brain cell growth which was reflected in improvements in their memory and learning. What is remarkable here is GPLD1 is made by the liver which affects brain functioning. This is remarkable, in that it shows a perfect example of liver-to-brain communication that to date, no researcher knew existed. The researchers than collected blood samples from human participants (*ages 66 to 78*) to see whether the GPLD1 protein would exert similar effects in humans. To their amazement, researchers discovered that GPLD1 levels were higher in the elderly participants that were physically active (>7100 steps per day) compared to those that were not physically active (sedentary) (<7,100 steps per day).

Reference
Blood factors transfer beneficial effects of exercise on neurogenesis and cognition to the aged brain. Horowitz AM, Fan X, Bieri G, Smith LK, Sanchez-Diaz CI, Schroer AB, Gontier G, Casaletto KB, Kramer JH, Williams KE, Villeda SA. Science. July 2020.

Summary
A protein that is generated by exercise restores age-related loss of memory and forms new brain cells. Older adults that exercise exhibit more of this protein in their body compared to sedentary adults. The results suggest that exercise may have a rejuvenating effect in addition to a preventative effect on aging. Future studies will hopefully uncover herbs and supplements that help the body's liver secrete GPLD1; thus taking these before exercise would exhibit a synergistic effect, greatly renewing brain function.

A formula that Relaxes and Renews the Muscles

Time to Feel Effects - Between 30 to 60 minutes after consumption.

This is a powerful formula that brings immediate relief to bursitis or other stiffness in the body. It is great for helping relax the nerves and muscles of the body. This could be why Roobios is such a powerful natural arthritis preventative.

Using loose Roobios herb or a tea, make a tea out of the roobios.

Next add between 3 and 4 drops of Roobios Extract and 2 drops of Reserveratrol Extract to the tea.

To make a Resveratrol extract, get the Resveratrol supplement in powder form and then make an extract out of it. This also allows the Resveratrol supplement to last 3 to 6 times longer, as the extract form of Resveratrol is much, much stronger than the supplement and it is better absorbed into the body. Sweeten the formula with honey or stevia extract. You can find out how to make your own Extracts in my best seller The Official Guidebook of How to Make Tinctures and Alchemy Spagyric Formulas.

Optional - If you want to enhance the effects even further, perform the Emerald Tablets, or similar Qi Gong or Tai Chi exercise. You can find out how to perform the Emerald Tablets Exercise by reading my book Deciphering Tablet Number XIII The Keys of Life and Death by Thoth the Atlantean (*recently revised in July 2019*).

Mega Strength Body Formula

This is a watered down version of the sulforaphane detox formula found in my recent anti-aging book (*published 2019*) The Official Guide to Reversing the Aging Process. Rashnya Herbs, Alchemy & Taoist Longevity Secrets. This formula is gentle enough to take up to 4 times in a row, with a 2 to 3 day break in-between, as it has an accumulative effect. It dries out and detoxes the body (*removing damp*), helping keep the immune system strong, but most of all it will greatly enhance the strength of the body. The formula also enhances the body's resistance to heat. Heat stress is known to be a contributor to the aging process and illness.

Sulphorane, a substance found in broccoli, is one of nature's most powerful pollution removers. Use this formula no more than 3 days in a row.

3 Drops of Willow Bark Extract (*is used to make aspirin*)
2 Drops of Lovage Extract (*abundant in Quercetin*)
3 Drops of Schizandra Berry Extract
2 Drops of Cinnamon Extract
2 Drops of Sulforphane Extract
1 1/2 teaspoons of Brewer's Yeast Powder

Take the above formula with flax seeds that have been soaking in water for 20 minutes or longer and add a little bit of honey. The following morning take 8 drops of Salacia Reticulata Extract to give the body an extra boost of energy and detoxification.

Neurocognition Protector Formula

Time to Feel Effects - Immediately

This formula is a great formula to take immediately after performing the Emerald Tablets, Qi Gong, Tai Chi or similar exercises. The reason why is because the body better absorbs nutrients into the body after these Chi generating exercises have just been performed.

1 apple sliced into 4 pieces with 1 drop of ormus on each side of the slice.
In 1/2 cup of water add the following-
A pinch of carnosine powder. Just open the supplement and remove the carnosine and sprinkle a small amount into the water. It takes 5 about 5 minutes to fully absorb into the water. (*Carnosine has no taste so don't worry about it tasting bitter*).
5 to 7 drops of Apple Peel Powder Extract. Apple peel powder is hard to obtain, but if you can get it and make it into an extract, it lasts for years and the apple peel powder also lasts a very, very long time.

NZT. Super Neurocognition Enhancer

Time to Feel Effects - 30 to 40 minutes after consuming

This is my favorite formula. I have used it for years to enhance my writing ability. I have called in the NZT Formula for short. This formula is so powerful, without any side effects, that the effects last up to 2 days after drinking it. It is a great formula to take before a test, exam or where long term mental endurance is necessary. This formula is unique in that many substances that enhance brainpower have numerous side effects such as headaches or fatigue. However, the "*coming down*" of this formula is very gentle. Besides enhancing mental strength, it also improves eye vision.

Bulk mix the below extracts and store in a cool dry place and add the drops to FO TI / Goji Berry Tea.

6 drops of butterfly pea extract
12 drops gotu kola extract
4 drops mucuna pruriens extract
3 drops rosemary extract
3 drops cordyceps extract

To supercharge the formula even further, before adding the above extracts, boil a pot of water with 8 finger nail sized pieces of Fo Ti root herb added to it and a pinch of Coptidis Rhizoma herb. Next remove from heat and add ½ a handful of goji berries and steep for 5 minutes. Next pour the tea into a cup or thermos and add 6 to 9 drops of the above NZT extract and take it with 1 Vitamin E capsule. You can either open the vitamin E capsule and pour it in or take it by mouth. *THIS IS KEY AS THE VITAMIN E ACTS AS A STRONG CATALYST FOR THE FORMULA*. It is also key when straining the Goji Berries that you press them firmly to extract the mini-seeds inside the Goji Berries as these tiny seeds are very potent antioxidants. If you don't have a strainer, than use a coffee filter to strain the herbs.

Optional
To strengthen the stomach, add between 5 and 8 drops of Black Bean Extract to the above formula, but no more or you will immediately flush your intestines out and really feel the cleansing effect. 0.5 drop of Coptidis Rhizoma extract.

A formula to Help Reduce Feelings of Depression
To ½ cup of water add the following extracts -
½ Drop of Syrian Rue Extract
Between 8 and 10 Drops of Banisteriopsis cappi extract

A Room Temperature Probiotic that needs no refrigeration

Time to Feel Effects - Immediately

Most probiotics are susceptible to heat. This is a great formula for "*on the go*".

2 drops Hawthorne berry extract
5 drops Salacia Reticulata
3 drops Astragalus extract
4 drops Elderberry

Notes on Elderberry -
Elderberry, one of nature's most powerful flu fighters, contains some extremely toxic substances that can become synergistic when mixed with other herbs. Use elderberry extracts sparingly and with common sense caution.
An Effective and Simple Exercise Recovery Formula

Time to Feel Effects - Immediately

Take this formula to bring fast relief to the body after intense work or exercise.

Walnuts that have been evenly sprinkled with grape seed extract powder
6 to 8 drops of Cordyceps extract
6 to 8 drops of Rhodioa Rosea extract
Regenerative / Summer Heat Stress Protection

Time to Feel Effects - 1 to 2 hours after performing physical exercise.

This formula only seems to work well when the outside temperature is above 86 degrees F or more and the body is exercising. It may be that it enhances the body's natural supply of antioxidants. It works extremely well when it gets very, very hot. I have achieved the very best results taking the formula before doing intensive exercise or a long bicycle ride in extreme heat. It actually feels like it regenerates the body via the exercise. It also protects against heat stress and is very good for strengthening the heart. This formula will also clear clouded eyes and strengthen them. This is because the high amounts of Vitexn found in the formula remove heat. In TCM bad eyesight is caused by the accumulation of heat, when combined with moisture in the air results in damp heat or "*steam*" which rises to the upper regions of the body and clouds the eyes. This formula also appears to help reduce feelings of a lack of energy. Instructions -

Bring a pot of water to boil with the following inside BEFORE the pot boils. This is because this formula contains numerous DNA herbs, that are always the hardest herbs to grind up. Hence, you can add these to the water before the pot boils to bring out more of the substances. Add to a pot of water and bring to boil the following herbs -

1 tablespoon of Mung Beans
5 to 9 Hawthorne berries (*these are always hard as rock and can be bought at a natural foods store or online*)
1/2 teaspoon of roobios tea
1/4 teaspoon of cat's claw
1 fingernail sized piece of Fo Ti root bark.

Optional -
After the water has boiled, remove from heat and steep. Next add the following extracts –

3 drops of reishi extract
2 drops of lovage extract (*quercetin*)
2 drops of hawthorne berry extract
4 drops of mung bean extract
3 drops of Ormus (*optional*)
Sweeten with honey

If you have not taken vitamin E capsules lately or your diet lacks vitamin E, be sure to take a vitamin E capsule with this formula, or you can cut open the top of the capsule and pour the vitamin E into the tea. Vitamin E is tasteless so you don't have to worry about a bitter taste like many anti-aging herbs have. Vitamin E also works extremely well for reducing dry skin in extreme heat.

Further Reading
Rhizoma Coptidis and Berberine as a Natural Drug to Combat Aging and Aging-Related Diseases. Zhifang Xu et al. Dec 2017.

The Brain Food Mix
This herbal combination boosts mental focus, mental energy and concentration.

1/2 Teaspoon of Rosemary
1/4 Teaspoon of Skullcap powder
1/4 Teaspoon of Cat's Claw
1/4 Teaspoon of Basil
1/4 Teaspoon Brazil Nut Powder
1/4 Teaspoon Mullein Powder
1/4 Teaspoon of Slippery Elm
1/4 Teaspoon of Astragalus
1/2 Teaspoon of Gotu Kola

1/4 Teaspoon of Cordyceps
1/4 Teaspoon of Jigoulan Herb or Ginseng
1/4 Teaspoon of Echinacea
1/4 Teaspoon of Ginkgo
1/4 Teaspoon of Bacopa (*optional*)
1/2 Teaspoon of Dan Gui Herb (*optional*)
1/2 Teaspoon of Papaya Enzyme (*optional*)
Alpha Lipoic Acid & N Acetyl Cyeteine - 1 Capsule or 1/4 Teaspoon (*optional*)

Take with warm water or a hot tea in the early morning or before strenuous mental activity. Works best when made as a tincture / extract which you can learn how to do in my book The Official Guidebook of How to Make Tinctures and Alchemy Spagyric Formulas. It is extremely important that you keep it away from damp environments. Does not store long as an extract, but works very well as a tea.

The SOD Mix
This is a long time favorite. Use it not only for energy, but to strengthen the knees. This is a great formula to help raise energy levels, relieve constipation and promote overall wellness. It is based on the ability to raise the body's Superoxide Dismutase levels naturally. Best taken early morning with 2 cod liver oil capsules 2 Vitamin C tablets and food.

Just under 1 1/2 Teaspoons of Brewer's Yeast
Just under 1 tsp Bromelain
Just under 1/2 tsp Teaspoon of Ashwagndha
Just over 1/4 tsp of Cumin Seed (*not black cumin*)
Just over 1/4 th tsp of FO-TI
Just under ½ of 1/4 tsp of Milk Thistle
Just under 1/4 th tsp of Creatine
Just over ½ of 1/4 tsp of Reishi

Just over ½ of 1/4 tsp of Ginger
Just over ½ of ½ of 1/4 tsp of Grape seed
Just over 1/4 tsp of Burdock
Just over 1/2th of 1/4 tsp of Cordyceps
Just over 1/4 th tsp of Basil
Just under 1/4 th Jiaogulan

Take with food during mid morning or just before or after a workout.

Stem Cell and Immunity Boosting Formula. The Overnight Rejuven Essence Formula
From the book: My Book of Stem Cell Longevity Formulas and Nutraceutical AntiAging Combinations.

An excellent formula for boosting the immune system and increasing energy levels and for developing strong and flexible bones; this formula is best taken before going to bed at night with honey. The following morning take the SOD mix mentioned earlier for optimal results. Combine the following and put into capsules:

On a late Friday afternoon or after an especially hard workout, take a food that is high in both niacin and melatonin. For example I use oatmeal seasoned with cinnamon. This is because oatmeal contains adequate levels of both melatonin and niacin.

After eating the meal, wait a total of 45 minutes to allow the niacin to fully be absorbed into the body.

After 45 minutes have passed, take a food that boosts the body's Superoxide Dismutase levels. I personally take a hot cup of Roobios Tea (*Aspalathuslinearis*). Physical exercise will also boost your body's Superoxide Dismutase levels (SOD) (*Free radical scavenging ability of Aspalathuslinearis in two invitro models of diabetes and cancer.Viduranga Y. Waisundaraa,*and Lee YianHoonb. January 2015*).

After another 45 minutes have passed, take the carnosine mix.

Natural Probiotic Formula
Simply put, this is a probiotic, but in an extract form. Add a few drops of this formula to plain Greek yogurt that has been mixed with cinnamon and flax seeds to give it an extra boost.

2 drops of Hawthorne Berry Extract
3 drops of Astragalus Extract
5 drops of Salacia Reticulata Extract
3 drops of Elderberry Extract
1 HN109 Probiotic Capsule

Optional -
1/2 Teaspoon of Jigoulan Powder (*or 3 drops of the extract*)
1 Alpha Lipoic Acid Capsule

The Carnosine Synergy Formula

Time to Feel the Effects - The following morning or 1 to 2 hours. It is not uncommon to feel the rejuvenative effects immediately after taking it.

This formula is an excellent recovery formula and it enhances knee strength. Take on a Friday night or during a full moon for maximum results.

Take the following capsules:

1 Milk Thistle Capsule
1,000 mg of carnosine
1 to 2 Vitamin C Capsules
Between 2 and 3 Cod Liver Oil Capsules (*Vitamin D*)
7,000 IU of Vitamin D3
200mg of Grape seed Extract Capsules
1 teaspoon of Brewer's Yeast (*B vitamins*)
2 to 3 tablespoons of honey

For an added boost, the below are optional -

Add the following extracts to 1 cup of spring water (alkaline)
4 drops of Elderberry Extract - note elderberry extract contains toxins, so it should be used with caution. If you feel uncomfortable taking it, then don't take it.

7 drops of Astragalus Extract
5 drops of Milk Thistle Extract (*liver stimulator*)
2 drops of Cayenne Pepper Extract (*catalyst*)
5 drops of Ormus (*enhances the absorption of all the aforementioned ingredients*)

The following morning take foods or supplements that repair the body's Myelin sheaths. Myelin sheaths strengthen the brain's neurons (*Pharmacogenetic stimulation of neuronal activity increases myelination inanaxon-specific manner. Stanislaw Mitew et al. Jan 2018*). I personally take berberine. Because the above formula stimulates the klotho gene, the body is better able to repair the myelin sheaths, which adds a major boost to the anti-aging properties of the formula.

Results are enhanced when taken with certain proteins such as anchovies or sardines. Other compatible foods include: honey, chicken soup, Parmesan cheese and black olives. Take with a few crystals of Himalayan Salt for an added boost. Lesser compatible foods include Cottage Cheese and Plain Greek Organic Yogurt (*Sweetened with Honey*). Taking Vitamin E the following morning also adds to the beneficial effects.

For maximum effectiveness, rub the upper shoulder and joints of the body such as elbows and knees and ankles with olive oil that has had gotu kola herb soaked in it for 30 days and exposed to the sun. The herb gotu kola and the nutrients in the olive oil exhibit major synergy. The olive oil infused with the gotu kola creates a more concentrated form of Olive Oil, meaning only a little is needed to cover the skin. Also excess olive oil rubbed into the body weakens the lungs, so it should be used sparingly.

Metal Chelation Mix
From my personal experience, this formula is very good at removing all types of allergies. An excellent formulation to chelate metals from the body. Take with 1.5 Tablespoons of Honey, 4 to 6 Cod Liver Oil Capsules and 2 Vitamin C Capsules for best results. Works best taken in early mornings and if you live in a large city metropolitan environment.

1/2 Teaspoon of Yerba Mate Herb
1/2 Teaspoon of Parsley Powder
2 1/2 Teaspoons of Brewer's Yeast
1 Teaspoon of Echinacea Powder
1/2 Teaspoon of Brazil Nut Powder
3/4 Teaspoon of Chili Powder
3 Bromelain Enzymes
1 Teaspoon of Garlic Powder

3/4 Teaspoon of Corriander
1/2 Teaspoon of Clove Powder
3/4 Teaspoon of Rosemary Powder
1 Teaspoon of Basil Herb Powder
A Pinch of Granulated Lecithin (*Optional*)
Between 2.0 and 10mg of Vitamin B6 (*Optional*)

A formula for rapid Recovery from Exercise
Rhodioa Rosea with Astragalus

A formula for boosting Sexual Endurance
Add 3 drops of each of the extracts of the following herbs to ½ cup of water: Jiaogulan, Schizandra Berry and Rhodiola Rosea

Chapter 18. Understanding the link between our Brain and our Immune System.

The Placebo Effect and Knee Surgery
Every year on average there are approximately 650,000 knee surgeries for arthritis of the knee, costing on average $5,000 per surgery. A study conducted by Dr. Bruce Moseley in 1996 discovered that participants given a fake sugar pill for a knee problem recovered almost just as well compared to a group that was given a real pharmaceutical pill. This study is key, showing that some pains in our body are psychological and that the power of belief can create healing in our body. Research has also discovered that the placebo effect is effective in one third of the human population (*The placebo enigma revisited. JMS Pearce. Emeritus consultant neurologist. August 2011*).

Reference
Arthroscopic treatment of osteoarthritis of the knee: a prospective, randomized, placebo-controlled trial. Moseley JB et al. Jan 1996.

Excessive Stress Contributes to Physical and Mental Illness
A lifestyle of constant chronic stress leads to plaque buildup in the arteries, contributing to the condition known as atherosclerosis. This is exasperated even further if the person's lifestyle includes a diet high in fats and a sedentary lifestyle.

A correlation exists between a stressful lifestyle and psychiatric illness, with those living a stressful lifestyle being more likely to be diagnosed with a medical condition or physical illness. (*Life Event, Stress and Illness. Mohd. Razali Salleh. Oct 2008*).

The Link Between Stress and Cancer
No scientific studies have found that a direct cause-and-effect relationship exist between the human immune system and one's chance of contracting cancer. Studies do exist however showing a link between stress, the body's suppression of natural killer (NK) cells and tumor development (*Psychologic stress, reduced NK cell activity, and cytokine dysregulation in women experiencing diagnostic breast biopsy. Linda Witek-Janusek et al. Feb 2014*).

Gratitude has been Scientifically Proven to Strengthen the Human Immune System
At a 4-day workshop conducted by Dr. Joe Dispenza in Tacoma Washington, the cortisol and IgA levels of 120 people were measured while the participants expressed positive emotions. Cortisol is a stress hormone; higher levels are bad for the body and deplete our energy. When cortisol levels rise, IgA goes down (*which is bad*). IgA is a powerful immune system protein. IgA is much better than a flu shot or immune system booster because it's totally natural.

During the workshop the participants were asked to move into elevated emotional states of joy, love or gratitude for approximately ten minutes. This was performed three times daily. The goal of the study was to see if one was able to bring balance to their immune system just by experiencing uplifting emotions. The study discovered that the participant's cortisol levels had dropped by three standard deviations, and that their IgA levels rose on average from 52.5 to 86 just by expressing these uplifting

emotions three times a day.
Reference
The Power of Gratitude. Dr. Joe Dispenza. Nov 25, 2016.

Making Your Gratitude List
The gratitude list (*Emmons and McCullough, 2003*) is when a person writes down three to five things they felt grateful for during each day. This simple and quick method has been proven scientifically to generate positive well-being (*the positive affect (PA)* (*Martínez-Martí et al., 2010*), happiness (*Mongrain and Anselmo-Matthews, 2012*) and life satisfaction. The gratitude list has also been found to reduce stress (*Kerr et al., 2015*) and depression (*Southwell, 2012*).

Another simple practice is just by simply writing letters of gratitude. When performed over a 3-week period, it has been shown to reduce depression and increase happiness and life satisfaction (*Toepfer et al., 2012*).

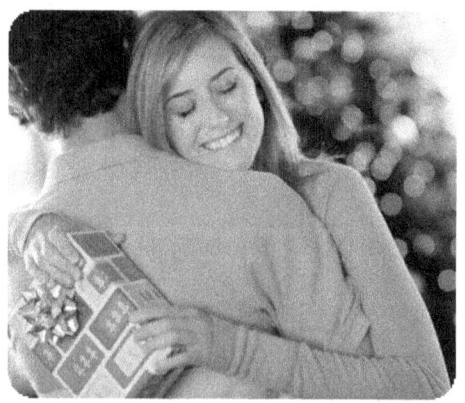

Summary
We don't need to turn to an over the counter pharmaceutical supplement or take exogenous substances to restore balance to our immune system. We have all the power we need to up-regulate our genes that govern our IgA. Hence, simply by experiencing the right emotions ten minutes a day, three times a day can restore balance to the immune system.

Stress is caused when one completely surrenders their power to the problem. Realize that problems are outside of you and should remain so. It is not what happens that determines the quality of your life, but instead HOW YOU RESPOND to circumstances that determines your future experiences.

Short term stress is good for the Immune System
Short term stress has been shown to be good for the immune system; however chronic stress has a significant long lasting effect on the immune system that ultimately manifests as illness. Long term stress has also been associated with ulcerative colitis, ulcers and even some cancers (*Life Event, Stress and Illness. Mohd. Razali Salleh. Oct 2008*).

Some studies have found that having a positive mindset reduces the alleviation of pain (*The Role of Positive Affect in Pain and its Treatment. Patrick H. Finan, Ph.D. and Eric L. Garland. Feb 2016*). This is good news for endurance athletes that may end up giving up due to the pain experienced in events or training. Having a positive mindset to overcome the temporary pain may make a difference between winning and losing.

Long term psychological stress has also been shown to alter the composition of the gut microbiota.

Reference
Galley JD, Nelson MC, Yu Z, Dowd SE, Walter J, Kumar PS, Lyte M, Bailey MT. Exposure to a social stressor disrupts the community structure of the colonic mucosa-associated microbiota. BMC Microbiol. 2014;14:189. doi: 10.1186/1471-2180-14-189.

How To Listen To Your Body's Subtle Messages To Enjoy Good Health

It is a now a scientific fact that excessive long term stress down regulates our genes, which causes chemical changes in the body which contribute to illness and dis-ease. This is because our cells were not meant to live in a stressful situation for extended periods of time. Hence, our environment influences our genes which create disease. Just by becoming more aware of something it reduces stress hormones and creates coherent brainwaves, which is why meditation can be used as a powerful healing tool.

The end product of experiences occurring in the environment cause emotions. Hence can our genes be signaled / controlled ahead of the environment by using positive / uplifting emotions? Research by Joe Dispenza discovered that participants (7,500 people) that took part in a meditation course for 4 days showed changes in 8 genes that lead to better health and a stronger immune system. So the answer is yes, changing genes through meditation can help one better cope with challenges in their environment.

A Harvard Study that was published in Psychological Science in 2007 found that a boring repetitive routine that was responsible for aches and pains was able to be transformed into something that is fun to do and in the process make one healthier. The study discovered that those who recognized their work as exercise experienced significant health benefits. The study involved approximately 100 room maids that worked in various hotels cleaning rooms. When they were instructed to think of the cleaning of their rooms as a form of outdoor exercise, they lost weight over a 4 week period, showed a reduction of body fat and exhibited lower blood pressure. All this just because they changed their AWARENESS of how they felt about what they did on a routine basis.
Reference

Mind-set matters: Exercise and the placebo effect. Crum, Alia J., and Ellen J. Langer. 2007. Psychological Science 18, no. 2: 165-171. 2007.

Restoring Order With Heart Coherence

Another effective method that restores order to one's being is practicing the new science of Heart Math. Heart Math is a technique where a person learns to breathe in and out through their heart. Heart Math benefits include; less stress, a reduction in anxiety and numerous other health benefits.

Reference
Treatment of Anxiety and Stress With Biofeedback. Christine Dunster. Sept 2012.

Using Heart Rate Variability to Improve Health

We are just starting to learn how to heal the body via the heart (*Angela J. Grippo 2017*). This is also known as 5th dimensional healing. This exercise utilizes Heart Rate Variability, which has been shown in numerous studies to help the body relax and release unwanted stress and tension.

1 -Go into coherence, expressing feelings of appreciation via Heart Math. You can use an EM Wave Meter to help you with this.

2. Once you have achieved coherence, picture a golden radiant glowing light around your body. Visualize this light restoring your body back to perfect health and harmony.

3. Next visualize yourself smiling into your heart.

4. Next visualize yourself smiling into all the cells of your body.

5. Next visualize yourself smiling into your immediate environment, such as your room, floor bed etc.

6. Next tune back into the golden revitalizing glow that surrounds your body and visualize your body in perfect health and harmony.

Repeat the above exercise 3 times over the course of 20 minutes or so, or until your body feels *'rejuvenated'* enough. For a much added boost, perform the exercise when your emotional biorhythm is peaking. This is because the exercise utilizes the energy of your heart. The heart is the generator of emotion in the body. Hence, you are using a peak period in your biorhythm cycle to tap into the energy of your heart and use it for healing /rejuvenation.

Chapter 19. Stimulus Check Information for United States Residents.

In March 2020, the United States experienced one of the most sudden and dramatic stock market declines in U.S. trading history. In just four market trading days, the Dow Jones Industrial Average dropped 6,400 points (an equivalent of roughly 26%). To help ease the burden of this sudden and unexpected shock to the economy, the Trump Administration introduced the Coronavirus Aid, Relief, and Economic Security (CARES) Act to act as a temporary safety net for those impacted by COVI-19. Also as of late October 2020, over 6 trillion dollars has been spent on various projects by the U.S. government. Examples include extended unemployment benefits, assistance to businesses and corporations and the like.

The CARES Act allows U.S. taxpayers or non- U.S. taxpayers to receive a payment of $1,200. For those filing jointly, they receive $2,400 (plus $500 per child). These payments are called Economic Impact Payments. These payouts gradually phase out for people whose incomes are above $75,000 Many stimulus checks were issued through direct deposits (directly into one's bank account).

Low-income individuals who do not usually file a tax return (with income below $24,400 for married couples and $12,200 for singles) are also eligible after filling out the "Non-Filers" tool application. For person's receiving Social Security benefits or are on Supplemental Security Income your stimulus check will automatically arrive into your bank account.

Where do I Sign up to receive my stimulus check?
To sign up, one must visit the IRS's "Get My Payment" page on the IRS.gov website and fill out an application form. The cut-off date to receive the first time stimulus check was late November 2020. However as of 2021, a new round of Stimulus checks has begun with the most recent being in March of 2021 for $1,400 for eligible individuals and households. An earlier payment was sent out in January of 2021 for $600.

How much stimulus money has been paid out so far?
As of August 28, 2020, the IRS issued approximately 153 million stimulus checks (approximately $269 billion). Officials overseeing the Coronavirus Aid, Relief and Economic Security (CARES) Act state that payments will cost a total of $292 billion through 2021.

The Official COVID-19 Guidebook of Published Studies, Resources, Supplements, Antivirals and TCM Herbs

Thank you for your interest in choosing a book outlining the clear facts about COVID-19 and the best herbs and methods currently used to fight the virus. Use the unique information in this text as a supplement for your COVID-19 arsenal The number of COVID-19 deaths is expected to increase in the coming months and possibly years. By having the right knowledge and information close at hand, you can have peace of mind you have some of the best information available to help you and your family defeat COVID-19 as well as being prepared ahead of time for when the next global pandemic unexpectedly strikes.

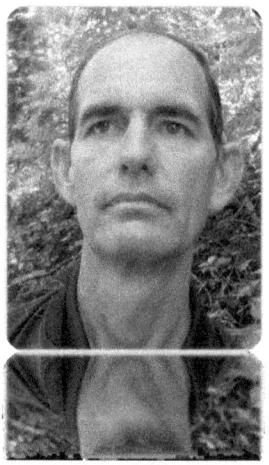

May you Enjoy a long and healthy life!!!!!

Scot Rauvers

Author

The Official COVID-19 Guidebook of Published Studies, Resources, Supplements, Antivirals and TCM Herbs

www.ingramcontent.com/pod-product-compliance
Lightning Source LLC
Chambersburg PA
CBHW060827220526
45466CB00003B/1001